CRITICALLY ILL

What is this and how do I use it? It's called a QR code. It allows you to Get In the Loop with me! Use a barcode scanner on your smartphone to unlock special content, videos and rewards from the author. As you read, scan the QR content (updated periodically) throughout this book for an even deeper, richer experience of Critically Ill.

About Frederick S. Southwick, M.D.

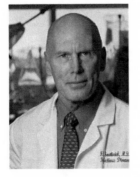

Dr. Southwick graduated from Yale College where he loved playing on the Varsity Football, Wrestling and Lacrosse Teams, and majored in educational psychology. He received his MD from Columbia College of Physicians and Surgeons, where he was an International Fellow and received the Edward J. Noble Foundation Scholarship. He trained in Internal Medicine and Infectious Diseases at the Boston City Hospital, and Massachusetts General Hospitals, and was an Assistant Professor at Harvard, followed by Associate Professor with tenure at the University of Pennsylvania, and in 1991 became the Chief of Infectious Diseases at the University of Florida.

He later was also appointed Vice Chairman for Research in the Department of Medicine. He has been an NIH funded investigator for over 30 years, studying how bacteria invade the host, and how white cells protect against bacterial invasion.

He also loves teaching, and has recently been focusing on the use of electronic interactive systems to encourage active learning by medical students. As a consequence of a family member's near death while being cared for in a University Hospital, Southwick became interested in the adoption of systems to improve frontline care, and the prevention of hospital errors. He has recently completed a year of study at the Harvard Business School as an Advanced Leadership Fellow, and is now the Projects Manager for Quality and Safety Pilot Programs for the UF & Shands Healthcare system.

About D.M. Treloar, ARNP, Ph.D

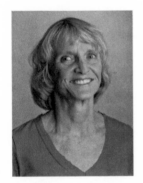

D.M. Treloar, ARNP, Ph.D has been a practicing nurse for 43 years, graduating from the Rutgers University College of Nursing in 1968. She has worked as a nurse in a public health, adult critical care, pediatric critical care and general medical surgical care. She completed her Ph.D in nursing in 1990, and ARNP in 1994, and is a tenured Associate Professor of the University of Florida. She serves as a preceptor for graduate nursing students, and now specializes in infectious diseases with a specific focus on HIV / AIDS. Most recently she has been promoting multidisciplinary rounds. She has worked closely with Dr. Southwick since 1994.

CRITICALLY ILL

A 5-POINT PLAN TO CURE
HEALTHCARE DELIVERY

Frederick S. Southwick, M.D.
with D.M. Treloar ARNP, PhD

PUBLISHING

For information on distribution rights, royalties, derivative works or licensing opportunities on behalf of this content or work, please contact the publisher at the address below or via email info@nolimitpublishinggroup.com.

COMPANIES, ORGANIZATIONS, INSTITUTIONS, AND INDUSTRY PUBLICATIONS: Quantity discounts are available on bulk purchases of this book for reselling, educational purposes, subscription incentives, gifts, sponsorship, or fundraising. Special books or book excerpts can also be created to fit specific needs such as private labeling with your logo on the cover and a message from a VIP printed inside.

No Limit Publishing Group
560 Carlsbad Village Drive Ste 202
Carlsbad, CA 92008
(760) 544-6070
info@nolimitpublishinggroup.com

This book was printed in the United States of America

DEDICATION

To my beautiful wife, Kathie Southwick, for her infinite patience and constant encouragement; to my parents, Ann and Wayne Southwick, for their lifetime of support and love; to my beautiful daughter, Ashley Southwick, for her heartfelt desire to always provide the best care to her patients; and to my son Peter, for his warm heart, boundless energy and loving companionship.

PRAISE FOR *CRITICALLY ILL*

"As Dean of the Harvard School of Public Health, I learned to respect the power and necessity of teamwork in delivering quality health care. *Critically Ill* is a gripping and personal account of the desperate needs for improving our health care system by an exemplary physician and caring human being. No one interested in improving how we as patients and families receive health care can ignore this iconoclastic book—or its key message that all of us must be part of the team required to improve health care delivery in this country."

—**Dr. Barry R. Bloom**, Harvard University Distinguished Service Professor, Dean of the Harvard School of Public Health 1998-2008

"Academic medical centers are faced with many complex and interdependent system problems that affect patient satisfaction and clinical outcomes. Curing our health care delivery system requires both top-down and bottom-up change. *Critically Ill* describes, in a manner that combines personal experience with research findings, a personal toolkit that will allow caregivers to improve the quality and safety of their patients' care."

—**Dr. David S. Guzick**, President, UF & Shands Health System

"Health care as never before requires adaptive leaders, that is, leaders willing to bring about true change. As Switzerland's Secretary of health I personally experienced the stresses associated with leading change. *Critically Ill* summarizes the key tenets of effective health care leadership, and will guide all leaders who aspire to transform how we care for patients."

—**Thomas Zeltner, M.D.**, Secretary of Health, Switzerland 1991-2009

"As a CEO who had to transform the culture of a major health care system, I applaud the blue print *Critically Ill* provides for organizing caregivers to bring about cultural change. This compassionate story of change is a recurring theme in US history, and the American can-do attitude permeates this book. Everyone who reads *Critically Ill* will be compelled to act."

—**Richard Pettingill,** President and CEO
Allina Hospitals and Clinics 2002-2009

"The Toyota production system (TPS), as applied to manufacturing, has been considered the most highly evolved management system in the world. Dramatic improvements in quality, safety and efficiency have been the result. We now understand that this same management system, adapted to healthcare, can demonstrate similar dramatic and sustainable results, improving healthcare quality, safety and efficiency. At Virginia Mason Medical Center in Seattle Washington this work has been achieving breakthrough results for over ten years. *Critically Ill* describes in very clear terms how care teams and individual caregivers can apply TPS in their organizations and practices to the benefit of their patients and communities. Our patients deserve at least the quality and safety that is applied to making automobiles and airplanes!"

—**Gary S. Kaplan, M.D.,** Chairman and CEO
Virginia Mason Medical Center

"With passion and personal stories, Dr. Frederick Southwick offers convincing evidence about the importance of teamwork in delivering positive outcomes. This timely book could make a big difference in transforming patient care."

—**Rosabeth Moss Kanter,** Harvard Business School Professor
and bestselling author of *Confidence: How Winning Streaks
and Losing Streaks Begin and End*

"Healthcare is normally portrayed as plagued by tradeoffs: quality at the expense of capacity, affordability at the expense of availability. Fred Southwick maps out an alternative for achieving improved quality, affordability, and availability. He does this, having faced a near catastrophe—the near death of his wife, Mary, due to egregious breakdowns in the delivery of care—and, at first, did what most of us do. He lashed out at the 'care providers' for absence of professionalism and compassion. But then Fred did something unusual. He analyzed the situation with clinical acuity and discipline normally reserved for patients, and he realized that the myriad process breakdowns would have overwhelmed even the most conscientious and heroic professionals. Befitting someone who picked a career dedicated to helping those unable to help themselves, he took his own personal discovery, documented it, and shares it with the rest of us to help understand how to plot a better course for healthcare to deliver on the full potential of the people it employs and the science it uses."

—**Steven J. Spear,** Senior Lecturer, MIT Sloan School of Management, Senior Fellow, Institute of Medicine, Author of *The High Velocity Edge*

"Reengineering Health Care provides a broad blueprint for how to improve patient care. However, the devil will be in the details. *Critically Ill* provides those details, and will allow caregivers to save lives by making the right decisions on the front lines."

—**Jim Champy,** Co-Author of *Reengineering Healthcare*

CONTENTS

ACKNOWLEDGMENTS

I would like to thank Mary Southwick Jones for allowing me to share our story with readers and audiences for nearly two decades; Harvard Advanced Leadership Initiative fellows Richard Pettingill and Fred Spar as well as fellow faculty member Dr. Nikolaus Gravenstein who read each chapter and provided incisive and honest comments that greatly improved the book's content; my sister Marcia Southwick who eagerly read each chapter and as a poet and creative writing professor provided encouragement and key ideas on how to improve the tone and readability of this book; the inspirational nurses who allocated valuable time out of their busy schedules for my interviews; my editor, Chris Snook, for his many creative suggestions; my fellow writer Jim Champy for his invaluable advice; and Harvard Professor Rosabeth Moss Kantor for her encouragement, action-oriented handouts, and outstanding leadership training.

In addition I would like to thank the Harvard faculty who assisted me in my courses: Professor Robin Ely, who so clearly and effectively taught "Leading Teams"; Professor Marshall Ganz and Ella Auchincloss, who lived and breathed the course "Organizing: People Power and Change"; Dr. Warner Slack and Dr. Don Berwick for organizing their insightful lecture series "The Quality of Health care in America"; and Maureen Bisognano, CEO of the Institute for Health Improvement (IHI) for her inspirational course "Improvement in Quality of Health Care."

Thank you also to Dr. David Guzick, CEO of UF & Shands HealthCare System, for his personal support and for enabling me to begin to implement many of the ideas I have described in *Critically Ill.* I appreciate my longtime nursing colleague Dina Treloar's enthusiastic assistance in my efforts to educate and empower the nursing community. And finally, I am grateful to the University of Florida Faculty Enrichment Opportunity Fund for providing me with the financial support to attend the Harvard Business School Advanced Leadership Initiative Fellowship and to write this book.

PREFACE

Our health care delivery system is critically ill, and despite calls from the Institute of Medicine and the remarkable efforts of organizations such as the Institute for Health Care Improvement, inefficiencies, errors, preventable patient injuries, and deaths continue unabated. Experts suggest that changes in our health care reimbursement systems are the key and that insurance reform will encourage and reward performance improvements. Certainly insurance reform will help. However, unless those on the front lines understand how to truly improve quality and safety, align their efforts through teamwork, and provide the leadership to change the way we do things, these conditions are unlikely to improve.

After analyzing these issues for more than twenty years and trying to implement improvement projects on the wards and clinics of our hospital, I realized the need for a book that addresses the fundamentals that each caregiver must learn in order to improve conditions at the bedside and in the clinic. When I was a boy, one of my favorite books was the Boy Scout Field Manual. This book described how to tie a square knot, how to build a campfire, how to pitch a tent, and how prevent water from seeping under the tent floor. These instructions and many more allowed me to safely enjoy camping in the woods. *Critically Ill* is a field manual for nurses and other caregivers, as well as for patients and patients' families. It is designed to guide the reader on how to safely provide and receive care. My hope is that this new understanding and these new skills will empower every reader to personally contribute to the improvement of care at the bedside and in the clinic, one treatment and one patient at a time.

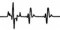

The first chapter of this book outlines my family's personal encounter with a dysfunctional health care delivery system, and the subsequent chapters describe how each aspect of Mary's care could have been improved. By asking why each step went wrong and how each aspect of her care could have been improved, this manual encourages the reader to develop new analytical skills for assessing and personally improving health care delivery. Each chapter begins with a series of guiding questions to encourage active reading. Throughout each chapter, key points are summarized to enhance the reader's learning, and individual patient cases are included to bring to life these key points. At the end of each chapter, a series of exercises is provided to encourage the reader to draw on past personal experience and to actively apply the principles he or she has learned.

The final chapter focuses on individual categories of nurse caregivers and provides specific action plans for each group. Many of these action plans are applicable to other caregivers as well. The best practices described throughout this manual will also provide patients and patients' families with an in-depth understanding of what constitutes ideal care. As educated health care consumers, they will be able to identify high-quality and safe caregivers and health systems. These newly acquired skills will enable both caregivers and patients to reduce preventable injuries and deaths.

As is true of all quality initiatives, this manual can and will be continually improved. I hope you, as an interested reader, will contact me with suggestions on how I can make this book better. As is stressed throughout my descriptions of quality initiatives, the reader should continually ask, what did I like about this book, and what could be improved?

—Frederick Southwick, M.D.
fsouthwick@gmail.com

−1−

WHO WAS CARING FOR MARY?

What can Mary's critical illness tell us about our health care delivery system?

Note to the Reader

As you begin this journey, you will find in the front of each chapter a handful of guiding questions to put the topic in the proper context as you begin to dive into the text. Please familiarize yourself with these questions at the outset of each section and revisit them after your immersion to derive the utmost value from this text, which is the culmination of twenty-plus years of study, practice, and successful application.

Guiding Questions

1. What conditions in Mary's case fostered preventable errors?

2. Who was to blame for the preventable errors that led to her admission to the intensive care unit?

3. How many people die from preventable errors in our health care system?

4. How can we fix our systems of care?

The events of Mary's hospitalization remain seared in my memory. Mary's illness took place in 1988; however, to this day I continue to find it hard to believe that a healthy thirty-three-year-old dance instructor and the mother of my two children could end up in the intensive care unit with less than a 10 percent chance of survival. How could this happen? The answers to this question reveal how a seemingly invulnerable young person can suddenly become extremely ill, and provide insights into how and why modern health care systems fail us to this day. I have recounted Mary's illness in three medical journals[1-3], spoken about these events at large gatherings of physicians, and described Mary's illness to my friends and acquaintances. Just like so many other victims of medical errors, my family and I have suffered. Like so many others, I became frustrated when I called out for help. I wondered to myself, *Does anyone really care?* We want the world to understand and to insist that our medical care systems improve and that caregivers prove through their actions that they truly care. I must warn you that Mary's story is an emotional one. But how could it be otherwise?

GATEWAY

http://bit.ly/tlVWwnJ

Mary's Story

As we sat in our chairs at the wake, Mary's mother talked about her husband, Tim. He had been a fireman when she met him. Handsome, funny, and a friend to so many—yes, Tim had been the life of the party. In his rich tenor voice, he had loved to sing "Danny Boy." She remembered the sad day when he fractured his arm while fighting a train fire. The doctors had to insert multiple pins to put his arm back together, and that spelled the end of his career in the fire department. That was the saddest day of his life, he had often

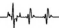

complained. But the good news was that he received a monthly disability payment for the rest of his life.

He soon secured a job at the Long Island Internal Revenue Service. Despite having only a high school education, he quickly moved up the ranks, and within five years was supervising four hundred employees. Tim cared about every employee. His charisma and empathy endeared him to all. His job supervising the processing of complex tax forms was often stressful. There also were always at least one or two employees with serious interpersonal problems. Not to mention the fact that he had the stress of raising six children. Tim loved his oldest daughter, Mary. She was the apple of his eye. Her deep brown eyes and sweet smile could melt his heart in an instant. Mary and her father had always been close.

Between family and work, Tim never had time to exercise, and he loved his eggs fried in butter, along with lots of bacon. He also loved to drink his evening beer as he sat in his recliner, watching sports on television. Over the years he steadily gained weight and developed hypertension. Tim was sixty-one when he experienced a sudden heart attack as he was walking to the commuter train. He died instantly. Mary was devastated. She had always been her father's favorite, and now he was gone. She cried and cried. I tried to comfort her, but for weeks she was sullen. I became concerned; I had never seen her like this.

In the hopes of improving her spirits, I arranged a family vacation to Florida. When I announced my plans, our children—Ashley, age five, and Peter, age eight—jumped up and down with glee.

"Dad, can we go to Disney World?" Peter asked.

Ashley followed with, "I can't wait to collect shells on the beach."

Mary gave one brief smile but then quickly retreated into the sadness of her loss. The sand and sun did improve Mary's outlook, but while on vacation both Ashley and Peter came down with sore throats. At the walk-in clinic, the rapid strep tests were positive, and both children were started on oral penicillin. Two days later Mary developed the same symptoms. I suggested she go the walk-in clinic. The children's visits had been very quick, but Mary refused.

"I am on vacation. Can't you just give me a prescription for penicillin? What's so great about you being a doctor if you can't even take care of your own family?" she complained.

I hesitated. I had always avoided treating my family, but Mary was just recovering from a profound personal loss, and her vigorous complaints indicated that she was finally returning to her old feisty self. I gave in and wrote a prescription for a ten-day course of oral penicillin.

Two days later we returned home. Mary's throat pain was resolving. I warned her that it was important to complete the full ten days of her penicillin. After four days of antibiotic treatment, her energy and spirits improved, and Mary returned to instructing aerobic dance at our local gym. I knew the exercise would continue to lift her spirits. When I returned from the hospital that evening, she raved about dance class. However, later in the middle of that night, Mary awoke complaining of sharp, burning, lightning-like pains on the bottom of her right foot. The pain failed to respond to aspirin.

We called our neighbor, an orthopedic surgeon, whose neurological exam revealed abnormal pain sensation as well as decreased muscle strength in the regions controlled by the right popliteal and posterior tibial nerves (the nerves behind her right knee responsible for pain sensation and movement of her ankle). Could she have injured her nerves during her previous day's dance routine? Mary denied any pain while dancing. Why would the onset of her pain be delayed for sixteen hours? My neighbor prescribed stronger pain medications, but her pain persisted.

On the seventh day of her symptoms, we sought the advice of a renowned academic neurologist who specialized in peripheral nerve injuries. He performed nerve conduction studies that revealed marked slowing of electrical conduction in the right popliteal and posterior tibial nerves, suggesting a peripheral nerve injury. Magnetic resonance imaging (MRI) of her right leg was within normal limits, revealing no evidence of trauma. Despite these MRI findings, the neurologist insisted that her nerve injury was the consequence of trauma brought on by dancing. I asked if any additional tests were warranted, and he assured us none were necessary.

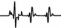

Upon our return home, Mary's pain began worsening. I phoned the neurologist, and he again refused to consider additional tests. He noted that he would be away at a research conference for the next week and suggested that I contact him when he returned. Despite several requests to his secretary that he see Mary, we never heard from or saw him again. I was disheartened and angered by his callous responses. After all, I was a fellow faculty member. I wondered how he treated his other patients.

On the ninth day, she developed blue painless hemorrhagic (blood-filled) lesions under her fingernails and on the sole of one foot. Later that day, her right ankle began to swell. I arranged an appointment with an internist at our medical center. She immediately ordered a venogram that revealed thrombosis (blood clots) in the right lower venous system and several superficial thigh veins. The internist recommended admission to the hospital but sheepishly reported that she was not on call and was already late for picking up her children at school. We felt abandoned—first the neurologist and now the internist. I had specifically requested this internist because of her excellent clinical reputation, but her other personal concerns clearly took precedence over Mary. I tried to understand. Physicians need to balance their lives and spend time with their families. But this was my wife!

Before heading to her car, the internist quickly phoned the on-call faculty physician, who arranged a hospital admission to the internal medicine service. The rotating intern, who had just begun his first month on the medical service, greeted Mary. He wondered out loud to the senior admitting physician whether someone with superficial thigh vein thrombosis warranted hospital admission. *Warranted hospital admission? Is this young man kidding?* I thought. I had a bad feeling about Mary's unusual presentation and its relentless progression. I pointed out the marked swelling of her ankle and the hemorrhagic lesions under her nail beds and on the sole of her foot. They thanked me for my observations but failed to consult dermatology or biopsy any of her lesions. I thought to myself, *They are ignoring my suggestions!* I kept quiet because I didn't want to interfere with their concentration. I realized I was supposed to be a supportive family member and needed to take off my doctor's coat.

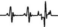

Admission studies revealed an elevated total peripheral white blood cell count of 18,000/μl (normal being 4,500–10,000/μl) with a greatly increased percentage of eosinophils (39 percent, with normal being 3.5 percent). Her total peripheral blood eosinophil count was twenty times higher than normal (7,021/μl, a normal count being less than 350/μl). Why did she have such extreme eosinophilia? The high number of eosinophils suggested a severe allergic reaction. Was she allergic to penicillin? When her foot pain began, I had told her to stop her penicillin. But unbeknownst to me, several days later, remembering my earlier instructions, Mary had restarted the antibiotic to complete her ten-day course of therapy. Or was she allergic to one of her pain medications? All of her previous medications were discontinued, and heparin (blood thinner) therapy was initiated to prevent further extension of the blood clots in her legs.

Except for her continued foot pain and a temperature of 102°F, all seemed well until the fifth day of her hospitalization. As we talked about Ashley and Peter, Mary suddenly grimaced midsentence. "Fred, I feel a little short of breath. My chest really hurts."

Upon further questioning, I learned that her pain was sharp, located on the right side of her chest, and much worse when she took a deep breath. We quickly called the medical resident, and as he examined Mary, she coughed up blood. I thought I was going to faint. Our nurse tried to comfort me. "Everything will be okay. You'll see." A lung scan confirmed my fears. Mary was suffering from a large pulmonary embolus. The blood clot in her leg had migrated up her right pulmonary artery and then broken apart. The resulting fragments had become trapped in the smaller peripheral arteries, cutting off the lung's blood supply, and caused a pulmonary infarction or lung tissue death. These events explained her severe chest pain and hemoptysis (coughing up of blood).

"Does she need an umbrella?" I asked the pulmonary specialist who had been called to assist in her care. This is a wire mesh device inserted into a large central vein (the inferior vena cava), to block the migration of additional clots from the legs into the lung.

"No, she doesn't need an umbrella. Her heparin doses were subtherapeutic," he said. (In other words, her blood had not been thinned as much as had been intended.) He frowned and then apologized. "I am really sorry about this. I can't tell you how many times these general internists screw up the heparin dosing. We are always having to bail them out."

This was the first time I learned that her partial thromboplastin time (PTT), a measure used to assess the ability of the blood to clot, had only increased to 41–42 seconds since admission. To effectively prevent the formation of new blood clots, the PTT should be maintained at levels of at least 70 seconds. Mary was now suffering the consequences of inadequate heparin therapy as she lay breathless and frightened in her bed.

I rushed to the senior physician's office. Why had Mary not received appropriate doses of heparin? He seemed unaware of any problems with her anticoagulation. He pointed out that he had delegated Mary's care to the senior medical resident and that I was welcome to speak to the resident at any time.

"Why don't you help with her care?" he suggested.

Being an academic physician myself, I understood the pressures her physician was experiencing trying to maintain his active clinical research program and at the same time manage patients on the medical wards. But this was my wife! I became frightened. Who was in charge? Additional sub-specialists were called to assist in Mary's care, but other than increasing her heparin dose, they recommended no additional therapeutic interventions. Her fever persisted, and her eosinophil count nearly doubled to 13,200/μl. This rise in eosinophils suggested to me that her allergic reaction was getting worse! The whole time I was thinking, *I am a doctor, and I can't get answers!* What if I had been a normal civilian who couldn't understand something was wrong?

On the eight hospital day, the senior medical resident called me. In a soft and hesitant voice, he reported that Mary had been complaining of a new type of chest pain and that her electrocardiogram (ECG) and cardiac enzyme blood tests had revealed a myocardial infarction—a heart attack! I couldn't believe it!

From a simple nerve injury, to blood clots in her legs, to a massive blood clot in her lungs, and now a heart attack.

Nausea, fear, anger, and sorrow all flooded me with an uncontrollable sense of urgency. I was afraid to leave Mary's bedside. I could no longer remain a passive observer. I reviewed Mary's medical chart. There was no mention of the subtherapeutic PTTs in the progress notes prior to her pulmonary embolus. The laboratory flow charts had not been filled out, and the chart did not contain much of the critical laboratory data generated in the last forty-eight hours. How could the consultants, much less the medical attending, possibly know what was going on? I spent the next two hours filling out the flow sheets in the hope that this act would assist our physicians in caring for Mary.

I discussed Mary's care with the floor nurses, and they commiserated. "We see this kind of thing all the time," one nurse volunteered. "We wish we could be of more help, but the doctors never ask our opinion about anything." The nurse softly and caringly wiped the beads of sweat from Mary's forehead as my wife restlessly squirmed in pain.

I slept on the floor in her room that night. I was afraid to leave her side even for one minute for fear another medical complication would arise. I felt helpless and frightened, like an observer on the side of the road, watching a Mack truck bearing down on Mary as she stood unaware in the middle of the road. I wanted to rush out and pull her from the truck's path, but I was tied to a tree and couldn't untie myself in time to save her.

I again spoke to Mary's physician. I pointed out that the rotating intern managing her case was overwhelmed. Clearly Mary's illness was beyond this young man's limited experience. Why hadn't he, as the senior physician, supervised her care more closely? My voice was strained as I tried to contain my anger. In my mind, he was to blame for all that had transpired, and I no longer trusted his ability to manage Mary's illness. I realized that additional dialogue would serve no purpose, and I transferred her care to a highly experienced cardiologist.

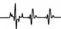

That night they convinced me to leave the hospital. As I lay in my bed at home, I kept going over each stage of her illness—the *ifs* and *why*s rushing through my head. I couldn't sleep and returned to her bedside at 2:00 a.m. Mary was sitting straight up in bed. She had an oxygen re-breather mask covering her face. She was gasping for air! I spoke to her nurse, who in a soft and concerned tone reported that two hours after I left the hospital, Mary had begun experiencing shortness of breath, and her chest X-ray now showed near complete opacification of her lungs. Opacification indicated that X-ray beams could no longer pass through her lungs because her lungs were filled with water rather than air. A normal chest X-ray would have shown dark areas where the lungs were located; however, in Mary's case, the lungs appeared almost completely white. Doctors sometimes called this "whiteout of the lungs," and I knew this was a very ominous finding. Her lungs had filled with fluid, and she was now drowning.

After seeing the chest X-ray, I burst into tears and ran from the room. I couldn't see Mary like this. The grief I felt cannot be explained. I too was hyperventilating. My head was pounding. I began whimpering, "My Mary. My dear Mary." I wondered if Mary died, what would I do? On my return home, my father tried to console me. Hysteria was not an option; we quickly returned to the hospital.

We found Mary again sitting upright in bed, agitated, confused, and breathless. She kept insisting that she needed to brush her hair. Her nurse tried to assist her, because each time Mary lifted the brush above her shoulders, her oxygen saturation dropped below 80 percent and an ominous warning alarm sounded. We knew that any further drop in her blood oxygen levels would be followed by seizures and/or death.

She whispered to me, "I am so tired. I can't last much longer."

"But, Mary, remember you have to help raise Ashley and Peter," I pleaded, and then I showed her this picture of our two children (see **Figure 1**).

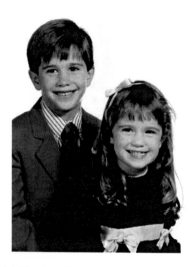

Figure 1. Peter (age 8) and Ashley (age 5)

"We love you and need you so much. You can't give up," I told her.

She nodded. We looked into each other's eyes as the anesthesiologist gave her a sedative and placed the breathing tube. I realized this might be our last communication in this world.

Despite assisted ventilation with high levels of end expiratory pressure (15 mm of positive end-expiratory pressure, which is used to improve oxygen exchange in the lungs) and administration of 100 percent oxygen, Mary's arterial oxygen levels were half of the normal values: PO2 levels at 45–50 mm Hg (normal being 95–100 mm Hg). She also became hypotensive, her systolic blood pressure dropping to 80 mm Hg. To maintain her pressure above this level required intravenous administration of dopamine, norepinephrine, and neosynephrine—agents that make the heart beat more vigorously and constrict blood vessels to raise blood pressure.

Our cardiologist began corticosteroids to lower her persistently high eosinophil levels. He suggested Mary could have been having a severe allergic reaction that was causing her eosinophils to attack her blood vessels and that all her clinical problems could have been caused by vasculitis (inflammation of the blood vessels).

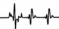

As I sat in the intensive care unit waiting room with my brother and Mary's mother, I expected someone to come in at any minute to tell me Mary was dead. I felt like I was sitting in the gallows and at any minute the hangman would arrive. As I waited I began thinking of all the wonderful things Mary had done for me. Mary loved to tell funny stories, and just like her father, she was the life of every party. I imagined that she was thinking of a joke at that very moment. That was Mary; she always looked at the humorous side of life.

I thanked Mary's mother for raising such a wonderful person. I realized I should be thankful for the ten precious years we had had together. Why did God want to take Mary from us? I had no answer. Was her father calling her to heaven? I realized I had to begin planning for our children's futures. How would I explain Mary's death to them? Should I move them closer to their grandparents?

Mary's ICU nurse came into the waiting room. I gritted my teeth. With gentle, empathetic expression of concern, she softly reported that there had been no change in Mary's clinical condition. With a tearful expression, she gave me a soft, comforting pat on the shoulder.

That evening a critical care specialist arrived. He had just returned from an academic conference. Rather than first going home to see his family, he had come directly from the airport to Mary's bedside to assist with her care. Together, the cardiologist, intensive care specialist, infectious disease specialist, and renal disease consultant remained at her bedside throughout the night, orchestrating her care. They discussed possible management alternatives and carefully planned her treatment. They knew there was no room for further error.

At 2:00 a.m. her kidneys were failing to excrete sufficient urine (less than a tablespoon per hour), and the renal specialist began placing an artificial hemofiltration unit to remove the excess fluid that had accumulated in her lungs. As he manipulated the catheter, Mary's heart suddenly stopped pumping. All electrical activity in her heart ceased. Her heart monitor showed a flat line in place of the normal sharp upward R wave of a heart in normal sinus rhythm. This is called an asystolic cardiac arrest, and it usually portends imminent death. As the alarms sounded, physicians and nurses from all over the hospital rushed to her bedside.

I bowed my head in prayer and squeezed the small wooden cross my brother had given me. My hands were sweating, and as I tightly squeezed this small object, my knuckles blanched. I held my breath as they pumped on her chest, and I thought as hard as humanly possible, *Please, Mary, don't leave me. We need you so much. Don't give up.* Her heart began beating again.

"Normal sinus rhythm," someone called out. I exhaled as I saw the normal EKG signal on her cardiac monitor.

The renal specialist quickly tried to readjust the hemofiltration catheter, and Mary suffered a second asystolic arrest. I knelt on the floor near her room. White-knuckled and sweating, I continued to grasp the small cross. I again saw the physicians pumping on her chest. My fear and hope shifted to sorrow and resignation. This had to be the end. My head again bowed, I desperately pleaded one last time, *Mary, you can't give up.* She didn't. Her heart monitor again showed a normal conduction pattern, and someone again yelled out in disbelief, "Normal sinus rhythm." Her heart had responded to atropine and isoproterenol—two drugs that could improve the electrical response of the heart.

An hour after her two cardiac arrests, Mary's urine output suddenly increased; she produced nearly four gallons of urine in less than 24 hours, and her lung function rapidly improved. I knew she would survive. As doctors often like to say, she had "turned the corner." Within five days, she was taken off the respirator. As they reversed her sedation, I rushed to Mary's bedside and gave her a kiss on the forehead.

In a light-hearted tone, her first words to me were, "Hey, why are you here? You make me nervous!" This sentiment reflected her last memories of my fearful expressions as I helplessly witnessed the seemingly unstoppable progression of her illness.

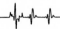

But now I could smile once again. I laughed as she continued to tell jokes and make light of our ordeal. After all, she had slept through much of her acute illness. But I knew that God, with the help of the physicians in the intensive care unit, had performed a miracle.

Over the next year Mary slowly but surely recovered. For three months she had difficulty walking, requiring that I carry her on my back upstairs to our bedroom. The pain from her nerve injury persisted for a year until the nerves fully healed. An expert immunologist who was consulted near the end of her hospitalization concluded that the likely cause of her illness was a very severe penicillin allergy that induced eosinophilia, peripheral nerve inflammation, and vasculitis. The administration of corticosteroids had been life saving. Fortunately once her corticosteroids were tapered, she suffered no relapse of her symptoms.

Our son, Peter, wrote this essay for his second grade class six months after Mary's return home:

> I like my mom when she acts very, very funny. We also like to go to malls together and go on upside-down roller coasters together. My mom likes me when I help her clean the house. I helped my mom when she came out of the hospital because she had a bad reaction to a medicine called penicillin when she was taking it for a cough. Then her nerve broke in her right leg, and she almost died. Mom always helps me when I have problems. When I broke my wrist, my mom drove all the way to the city just for the X-ray. My mom loves me even when I am grumpy.
>
> —Peter Southwick, 8 years old

Peter and Ashley were able to grow up with the nurturing care of their mother; they have now graduated from college and are establishing their careers. Mary and I did not beat the statistics when it came to staying together. However, we are both happily remarried, and life has continued to move on. However, the memories of Mary's near-death experience will be with us forever.

Why Is Mary's Case Important to the World?

Just as Mary, my children, and I will never forget these events, thousands and thousands of other families have similar unforgettable stories. In many cases they are not as lucky as we were. One out every ten patients will suffer from an error while hospitalized[4, 5], and the incidence of preventable deaths ranges from 14–27 percent of all in-hospital deaths. After my first paper describing Mary's illness was published in the Annals of Internal Medicine[1], I received more than ninety personal letters from concerned physicians empathizing with her story. Many letters described similar experiences. Anger, sorrow, remorse, and loss ran through each story. And Mary's case illustrates the personal toll of medical errors.

Mary's case also illustrates the financial toll of medical errors. As shown in **Table 1.1**, because of the multiple missteps and delays, rather than requiring a four-day admission on the general medical wards—the typical duration of hospitalization for thrombophlebitis (cost of care $16,280)—Mary required twenty-two days of hospitalization, with thirteen of those days being in the ICU (cost $92,209). The cost of her care was nearly six times what it should have been if the systems and caregivers had been functioning properly.

Table 1.1 Estimated cost of Mary's care

Cost of Mary's Actual Hospitalization	
Seven days general medicine floor (heparin, laboratory tests, ventilation-perfusion scan, oxygen, etc.)	$23,144
Thirteen days MICU (respirator 7 days, hemofiltration, IV medication, cardiac catheterization, two cardiac arrests, etc.)	$61,342
Two days general medical floor (ultrasound, blood tests, chest X-ray, nerve biopsy, etc.)	$6,280
Total for hospital episode:	**$92,209**
Costs of Mary's Hospitalization if Error-Free	
Four days general medical ward for thrombophlebitis	**$16,440**

Each year in the United States, there are an estimated 44,000–98,000 deaths caused by preventable medical errors, which is a higher death rate than for motor vehicle accidents (43,000 deaths a year)[6]. Other studies suggest the death rate associated with medical errors is considerably higher[7, 8]. The estimated annual total cost of healthcare associated preventable deaths and injuries in the United States is $17–29 billion[6].

Despite the fact that these facts have been widely publicized for over a decade, the grim statistics have not improved, and cases such as Mary's continue unabated. Despite the aggressive institution of safety programs in the majority of hospitals, there has been no significant reduction in harm to our patients. For example, a large group of North Carolina hospitals discovered that one out of every four of their patients was harmed in the hospital. Five years after the adoption of nationally recognized safety programs, analysis of patient outcomes has revealed that these same hospitals continue to harm one out of four patients[9].

Systems engineers and physicians focusing on safety now understand the nature of human error and have developed exciting design improvements that take human behavioral factors into account. Innovative programs that can reduce infections and patient falls, as well as surgical and medication errors, are available and have been implemented in single institutions and in small regions of the country. However, these practices have not spread uniformly, attesting to the difficulty of instituting the changes necessary to make our patients safe.

Why is the implementation of quality and safety programs so difficult? One major reason is a lack of motivation on the part of caregivers and patients. Humans often fail to respond to statistics because statistics are abstract, and personal experience is a much more powerful driver of behavioral change. A careful analysis of Mary's case can teach each of us about safety and quality in health care. By truly understanding what happened to Mary and why, each of us can contribute to the solutions rather than continuing to accept the present conditions on our wards and in our clinics.

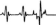

Who Is to Blame?

Should We Blame Physicians and Nurses?

For nearly fifteen years, I solely blamed Mary's illness on the physicians who cared for her, including myself. At the time of my first paper describing her case, national organizations were also emphasizing individual physician accountability. The American Board of Internal Medicine sponsored Project Professionalism[10], and the nursing profession at that time was also focused on individual professionalism[11]. No one would disagree that each physician and nurse should strive to achieve his or her professional goals. And individual accountability did play a critical role in the care that Mary received. Certainly the neurologist who first saw Mary lacked professionalism and should have been censored and counseled.

As I look back on these events with a less emotional eye, I now realize that the first inpatient senior physician did care, but he had appeared uncaring because he had failed to prioritize his many duties to free sufficient time to fully concentrate on Mary's illness. Mary's consulting subspecialists went to great lengths to assist in her care and certainly should not be criticized for lack of effort. Our nurses expended great effort on our behalf; however, the lack of effective coordination between physicians and nurses resulted in ineffective care. I now realize that the solution cannot be to simply insist that the physicians and nurses try harder and pay more attention.

My conclusion agrees with the teachings of patient safety and quality experts: *We now know that individual physicians and nurses simply working harder and being more focused are unlikely to prevent cases like Mary's from recurring.* Over the past two decades, the complexity of health care has progressively increased. As a consequence, no single individual can manage the large amounts of data or coordinate the large number of care providers required to effectively manage each patient's illness. Although individuals contributed to Mary's downward hospital course, it was dysfunctional systems that were primarily responsible.

In addition to victimizing patients, our dysfunctional systems often place nurses in compromising conditions. I never blamed the nurses who cared for Mary because they lacked any authority to improve Mary's care. Throughout Mary's hospitalization they shared their concerns with me. They were forced to look on as horrified bystanders as physicians mismanaged Mary's case. Like me, they felt helpless in the hierarchical structure that prevented them from questioning physicians. They knew all too well that, in the prevailing culture, if a nurse made suggestions for improving Mary's care, physicians would interpret their actions as disrespectful. If the nurses had aggressively advocated for changes in Mary's care, they would have been disciplined.

Should We Blame the Consumer?

Patients have difficulty getting the true facts about our health care system, making it almost impossible for them to act as educated consumers. Thirty-second sounds bites and mischaracterizations of the facts have created fear and misunderstanding. Who wins under these conditions? At the national level, one of the primary goals for everyone should be to establish a rational and factual basis for decisions about population health and patient care. Shrill dialogue and simplified black-and-white mischaracterizations have no place in life and death decisions. Remember, the claim that news reporting is "fair and balanced" doesn't make it so.

When it comes to understanding health care, patients and the lay public will need to avoid most mass media sources and turn to objective, neutral resources such as *Consumer Reports*, other nonprofit news sources, and peer reviewed medical journals to obtain the truth. Consumers need to realize that their lives are at stake. They need to insist on a dialogue that is based on objective facts derived from economic, business management, and biomedical research. That is the only way to improve the health status of both the haves and the have-nots.

Should We Blame Our Politicians, Pharmaceutical and Health Equipment Manufacturers, and Health Insurers?

Many politicians claim that the United States provides the best health care in the world. Are they lying? When it comes to "rescue medicine" such as the heroic treatment Mary received in the ICU, we are indeed the best of the world. And when it comes to cutting-edge technology and sophisticated new procedures, we again are the best in the world. Our pharmaceutical industry and health care equipment manufacturers have succeeded spectacularly. They have clearly fulfilled their mission. And the health insurance industry has tried valiantly to reduce the costs of care by closely monitoring physicians' decisions and in some cases partnering with physicians. However, costs continue to escalate.

Despite the ever-increasing costs of per capita of U.S. health care, routine and preventative care are not improving in quality. In fact, just like the care physicians provided for Mary in the early phases of her illness, standard care is woefully deficient. Adult patients in the United States receive only about 55 percent of the therapies and preventative measures widely acknowledged as the standards for care[12]. The U.S. health care system is presently only ranked thirty-seventh among industrialized countries, just behind Costa Rica and just ahead of Slovenia and Cuba[13, 14]. And we have achieved this low ranking despite outspending all other industrialized countries twofold.

We must all ask ourselves if it is worth spending more than twice as much per capita on health care (more than $7,500 per capita) as most other industrialized nations ($3,000–3,500 per capita)[15] while having so little to show for it. In the business world, such poor efficiency would inevitably lead to bankruptcy. However, rather than going out of business, the U.S. health care system simply consumes a greater and greater percentage of our nation's gross domestic product (GDP). The percentage of our GDP devoted to health care is now estimated to be 17.6 percent, and shows no signs of decreasing[16].

Our nation clearly has the know-how, the initiative, and the resources to create the best health care system in the world. We just have to make up our minds and commit to not only achieve technical excellence but also to achieve excellence in the delivery of safe, efficient, and high-quality care.

Conclusion About Who Is to Blame

No one person or one of group of leaders can be blamed for the present state of our health care system. *We are all to blame.*

Sadly, in many health centers, the systems of care have not significantly improved over the past two decades, and it is well recognized that when there is change, there will be winners and losers. Unfortunately, when it comes to changing the hierarchical culture and fragmented systems of care in our hospitals and clinics, the defenders of the status quo continue to hold on to power. Mary's experience and the suffering of so many other injured patients clearly show us that the status quo should no longer be acceptable.

How Can We Prevent Another Case Like Mary's?

Mary's illness should be viewed from a systems perspective in order to identify strategies for improvement and to prevent other cases like Mary's. There were six stages of Mary's illness and seven different categories of systems defects (see **Table 1.2**).

Table 1.2 Stages of Mary's illness, actions, errors, and proposed solutions

Stages	What happened	What went wrong	What should have happened
1: Family member prescribed penicillin (PCN)	He diagnosed Streptococcal pharyngitis and prescribed PCN.	He missed family history (FH) of severe PCN allergies and obtained no throat culture.	Physicians should not treat family members; seek outside care.
2A: Outpatient neurology visit	Neurologist diagnosed a damaged nerve caused by physical injury.	He failed to determine underlying cause of her neuritis and ignored the negative MRI.	Care protocol: Recent meds, FH of PCN allergies, blood smear and white blood cell count.

Stages	What happened	What went wrong	What should have happened
2B: Discharge from neurology without follow-up	Neurologist left for a conference.	There was no handoff to a neurologist; Mary's care had to be transferred to an internist.	Handoff to neurologist would have maintained focus on the primary problem.
3: Outpatient internal medicine clinic	Internist left to pick up her children.	There was a rushed handoff to a third physician who was unfamiliar with Mary's case.	A physician should have been appointed for person-to-person sign-outs and admissions.
4A: Admission to general medical ward	Heparin was underdosed.	Mary suffered a pulmonary embolus.	Protocol ensures correct heparin dosing.
4B: Ward team management	Head physician was unaware of heparin error.	There was poor team communication and teamwork.	There should have been clear team communication protocols.
5: Myocardial infarction (heart attack)	Multiple organs were affected, indicating a multisystem disease.	Each consultant focused on one organ system (vertical care).	Opinions of consultants should have been integrated.
6. Cumulative errors	Mary was admitted to ICU.	Mistakes led to her worsening illness.	The above corrections would have prevented admission to the ICU.

At the first stage of her illness, I inappropriately prescribed a medication—penicillin—without performing a full history and physical. I failed to elicit Mary's very strong family history of penicillin allergies. In fact, following penicillin administration, one of Mary's brothers at age four developed temporary quadriplegia (paralysis of all four limbs) and a desquamative (peeling) skin rash; her sister developed mouth ulcers and a skin rash; and her father developed a desquamative skin rash.

At the second stage of Mary's illness, the neurologist ignored the normal result of her MRI and falsely attributed her nerve injury to trauma. Most disappointing, he failed to hand off Mary's care to a fellow neurologist when he left for an out-of-town conference.

At the third stage, our internist focused strictly on Mary's thrombophlebitis (blood clots in her legs) and failed to identify the neuritis (inflammation of her nerves) and hemorrhagic skin lesions (dark red skin lesions containing blood) as key components of a systemic illness (an illness that involved many organs). Furthermore, this internist very quickly and superficially handed Mary off to a third physician. She was more focused on her family obligations than her obligations to Mary.

The physicians' failure to use a heparin dosing protocol in stage four resulted in the underdosing of Mary's heparin, and nurses were not empowered to manage what should have been a routine medication administration. Furthermore, although they were aware of the underdosing of her heparin, the nurses were fearful of communicating this problem to the physicians. There also was no system for integrating the input of the multiple subspecialists who saw Mary. There were no clear expectations, job descriptions, or clearly defined customer-supplier relationship for the many care providers who were trying to help Mary during her initial hospitalization.

I've thought about the critical errors and misjudgments that led to Mary's near death for more than twenty years, and I now understand that there are many successful systems that perform at very high levels. These high-performing systems exist in team sports, manufacturing, and commerce. Why couldn't hospital systems adopt these widely practiced principles? By adopting the best practices from successful manufacturing and athletic teams, medicine does not need to reinvent the wheel, and Chapter 2 of this book will examine how Toyota, Southwest Airlines, and Publix, as well as University of Florida athletic teams, have reached the very top of their respective competitive arenas. An understanding of these principles would have encouraged improved patient handoffs, the use of protocols, and improved nurse-physician and ward team-consultant working relationships.

A specific heparin protocol combined with nursing and pharmacy second checks could have provided three stages of quality assurance and prevented the underdosing of heparin. Chapter 3 discusses the concepts of normal variation and human error, the importance of reliability, the many tools available to prevent errors, and the great need to improve our systems of care to protect caregivers from making, and our patients from suffering the consequences of, human errors. If the physicians and nurses caring for Mary had embraced the tenets of patient safety outlined in this chapter, the story of Mary's encounter with a university medical center would have been a tale of relatively simple, ordinary procedures leading to a positive outcome, and I would not have written this book.

But none of these conditions were in place, and as a consequence, Mary developed a large pulmonary embolus (a large blood clot from her legs that migrated to her lungs). This was followed twenty-four hours later by a heart attack, ushering in the fifth stage. Her consultants were following her very closely as she became sicker and sicker, and in their notes they expressed their concerns. The hematologist noted that the high number of eosinophils in her blood might be attacking her blood vessels and could explain her heart attack. He suggested that corticosteroids be started. However, the senior physician failed to act. The input from the hematologist, pulmonologist, neurologist, orthopedic surgeon, and cardiologist were never fully integrated to derive a unifying diagnosis. It was only in the sixth and final stage of her illness that a unifying diagnosis was made and corticosteroids initiated. However, the accumulation of errors and delays left Mary near death, and it was only through remarkable heroics, careful coordination, and expensive interventions that she was rescued.

Her initial hospital admission—the fourth stage of Mary's illness—in many ways represented the most disastrous stage. As will be discussed in Chapter 4, the physicians that admitted Mary were a working group rather than a working team. If the rounding team caring for Mary had included her bedside nurses, and if the physicians had actively communicated with them, the nurses would have likely shared their concerns about Mary's sub-therapeutic partial prothrombin time (PTT). As a second check, the pharmacist could have reviewed the heparin infusion rate and also noted the low PTT value. Each physician worked as an independent caregiver, and no one caregiver proved capable of managing the complexity of Mary's case or coordinating the input of the multiple consultants. As a consequence, no one was able to generate a unifying diagnosis or create an effective treatment plan. The individual caregivers simply watched helplessly as Mary's condition deteriorated.

In addition to lacking the skills to create a true team, the senior physician who cared for Mary during the fourth stage of her illness ignored well-established leadership principles that will be discussed in Chapter 5. He failed to establish Mary's care as his top priority and instead was multitasking, trying to perform his administrative, research, and patient care duties simultaneously. He also failed to take charge and act on the information he had received from his consultants. The senior medical resident demonstrated poor leadership in his supervision of his intern. And the nurses were discouraged from leading because of the steep hierarchical power gradient that existed in the hospital. To bring about true changes in these conditions, we will need adaptive nursing leaders that effectively challenge the status quo and change how doctors and nurses work together. Without adaptive leaders, efficient systems of care, robust safety tools, and effective teamwork cannot flourish.

The prevailing behaviors of the health care providers involved in Mary's care revealed a dysfunctional set of cultural norms that interfered with the adoption of a true systems approach to patient management. The physicians who first saw Mary felt comfortable quickly dropping her from their care, and the senior physician who first cared for Mary devoted little time or energy to her care. These actions suggested that they viewed patient care as less important than research or family obligations. The prevailing culture also tolerated other dysfunctional norms, including the practice of avoiding communication with bedside nurses and the tradition of acting as lone practitioners.

These behaviors reflected deep-seated implicit values that were not focused on the patient but rather somewhat paradoxically on the needs of the physicians. Early in their medical training, physicians are taught the primacy of the patient, the importance of self-sacrifice, and the Hippocratic credo of "do no harm." However, in a culture where research is primarily rewarded and in a society where family and self-fulfillment are emphasized, these important values can progressively decay. Chapter 6 will describe a constellation of proven methods that directly address the values and motivations of an institution, and these approaches can achieve ground-up cultural change. Before quality and safety programs can be implemented, many of our health care systems will require a cultural makeover.

Physicians, nurses, administrators, health professions students, and patients all need to develop a deep understanding of manufacturing and athletic systems, human error, and the principles for improving safety, teamwork, adaptive leadership, and organizing people to bring about cultural change. However, it is impossible to address all of these divergent constituencies in a single book. Therefore, I have chosen to focus on nurses and nursing students in *Critically Ill*.

Why? First and most importantly, based on more than thirty years of personal observation, I have found that nurses are the caregivers who most consistently focus on the patients' needs and interests. They are at the bedside the majority of each shift, where they personally help each patient cope with illness. As we found in Mary's case, nurses empathize with their patients' suffering.

Second, unlike most physicians who have a monetary interest in increasing the amount of care they provide through procedures and tests, nurses have no conflict of interest. They are paid a fixed salary and can objectively serve as patient advocates. When it comes to deciding patient care policies, in my view, nurses should have the final say.

Third, nurses physically care for their patients. They hand out the medications, manage the intravenous solutions, supervise physical therapy, and advise their patients on how to manage their illnesses. When the customer-supplier relationships are dysfunctional, nurses are unable to carry out their vital tasks, and the patient suffers. When systems are defective, the likelihood of errors increases, and because nurses provide the direct care, they are at greatest risk of inadvertently harming their patients. The guilt and remorse associated with serious errors causes nurses, as well as patients, great pain and suffering. In defective systems, nurses are in danger of becoming second victims.

Finally, nurses represent the single largest group of caregivers, and they are often socially engaged and possess extensive networks. They are the constituency that has the greatest potential to bring about cultural changes in our clinics and hospitals.

After reviewing the five-point plan to cure health care delivery, the final chapter will provide action plans for how nurses, nurse practitioners, nursing administrators, and nursing students can personally improve how health care is provided in their hospitals and clinics. All caregivers, but particularly nurses, need to think of Mary's story each time they identify a system defect, a condition likely to breed an error, an example of poor teamwork, an ineffective leader, or an unhealthy cultural norm. Once they identify these problems, rather than simply shaking their heads and throwing their hands up in disgust, the final chapter will describe how they can apply the skills and understanding derived from Chapters 2–6 to work effectively with physicians, administrators, and patients to correct each problem they encounter.

As Mary's case so clearly illustrates, families and patients see health care professionals and the system as a single entity; if the systems of care are flawed, even proficient and compassionate nurses can be perceived as inept and uncaring. My hope is that the remembrance of Mary's story will motivate nurses to devote their energies not only to improving their personal skills but also to improving our care delivery systems. By improving our systems one small step at a time, we can achieve the quality of health care that we all aspire to provide and the quality of care each patient expects and has the right to receive. Yes, each of us can make a difference!

References

1. F. Southwick. 1993. Who was caring for Mary? *Ann Intern Med* 118 (2):146-148.

2. F. Southwick. 2001. Who was caring for Mary? 1993. *Obstet Gynecol* 98 (6):1140-1142.

3. F. S. Southwick, and S. J. Spear. 2009. Commentary: "Who was caring for Mary?" revisited: a call for all academic physicians caring for patients to focus on systems and quality improvement. *Acad Med* 84 (12):1648-1650.

4. L. L. Leape. 2010. Personal Communication.

5. R. W. Dubois, and R. H. Brook. 1988. Preventable deaths: who, how often, and why? *Ann Intern Med* 109 (7):582-589.

6. Linda T. Kohn, Janet Corrigan, Molla S. Donaldson, and Institute of Medicine (U.S.). Committee on Quality of Health Care in America. 2000. *To err is human : building a safer health system*. Washington, D.C.: National Academy Press.

7. C. Zhan, and M. R. Miller. 2003. Excess length of stay, charges, and mortality attributable to medical injuries during hospitalization. *JAMA* 290 (14):1868-1874.

8. J. S. Weissman, E. C. Schneider, S. N. Weingart, A. M. Epstein, J. David-Kasdan, S. Feibelmann, C. L. Annas, N. Ridley, L. Kirle, and C. Gatsonis. 2008. Comparing patient-reported hospital adverse events with medical record review: do patients know something that hospitals do not? *Ann Intern Med* 149 (2):100-108.

9. C. P. Landrigan, G. J. Parry, C. B. Bones, A. D. Hackbarth, D. A. Goldmann, and P. J. Sharek. 2010. Temporal trends in rates of patient harm resulting from medical care. *N Engl J Med* 363 (22):2124-2134.

10. J.D. Stobo, J.J. Cohen, H.R. Kimball, M.A. Lacombe, G.P. Schechter, and L.L. Blank. 1995. Project Professionalism. Philadelphia, PA: American Board of Internal Medicine.

11. B. K. Miller, D. Adams, and L. Beck. 1993. A behavioral inventory for professionalism in nursing. *J Prof Nurs* 9 (5):290-295.

12. E. A. Mcglynn, S. M. Asch, J. Adams, J. Keesey, J. Hicks, A. Decristofaro, and E. A. Kerr. 2003. The quality of health care delivered to adults in the United States. *N Engl J Med* 348 (26):2635-2645.

13. Who. 2000. World Health Organizaiton Assesses The World's Health Systems. *WHO Press Release, June 21, 2000.*

14. C. J. Murray, and J. Frenk. 2010. Ranking 37th--measuring the performance of the U.S. health care system. *The New England journal of medicine* 362 (2):98-99.

15. Oecd. 2010. Organisation for Economic Co-operation and Development Health Data.

16. CMS, Centers for Medicare and Medicaid Services. [cited October 9, 2011]. Available from http://www.cms.gov/ NationalHealthExpendData/25_NHE_Fact_Sheet.asp.

Chapter 1 Exercises

1. Do you or a close acquaintance know anyone who suffered from preventable complications in the hospital?

    a. Describe what happened.

    b. Why did it happen?

    c. How could their problems have been prevented?

    d. Do you believe this episode should be blamed on an individual, or should it be blamed on the system?

    e. Do you feel your nurse was an effective leader who advocated for your care, or was she simply obediently following the instructions of the physician?

2. Describe your own visit to a clinic or a hospital.

    a. Were the health care personnel friendly and focused on your needs?

    b. Did you feel that the personnel worked well together?

    c. Was the workflow well organized?

    d. Did you witness any mistakes or oversights?

    e. Do you have any suggestions for how your visit could have been improved?

3. Describe an experience at your favorite store.

    a. Were sales people friendly and focused on your needs?

    b. Did you feel that the personnel worked well together?

    c. Was the store well organized?

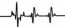

d. Was your sales person prompt and helpful?

e. Did you witness any mistakes or oversights?

f. Do you have any suggestions for how your store experience could have been improved?

-2-

INDIVIDUALS MAKE PLAYS; PLAYBOOKS WIN CHAMPIONSHIPS

What Can Industry and Athletics Tell Us about Mary's Care?

Guiding Questions

1. What is a push-manufacturing business model and what can this model tell us about the marked differences in health care costs in different regions of the United States?

2. How can we apply the 80/20 rule to the care of our hospitalized patients?

3. How do we create conditions that reduce waste and improve workflow in our health care systems?

4. What is meant by work-around solutions and why should we avoid them?

5. How can caregivers improve the coordination of patient care based on principles derived from the airline industry?

6. How do we achieve and reward exceptional service to our patients?

7. What do championship athletic teams have in common with high-performing industries, and what lessons do they provide for health care?

Lost Opportunities

Two physicians—the neurologist and the first internist—quickly released Mary from their care. In the case of neurologist, he left for a meeting and never contacted us again, despite repeated requests. A Toyota employee would say he had "disrupted the value stream" while a football coach would be screaming "Fumble!"—one of the most dreaded adverse events in football. Mary's care was not handed off to another outpatient neurologist, and therefore she lost the potential value of a neurological specialist as her illness evolved.

During the later phase of Mary's hospitalization, another neurologist was consulted, and this second neurologist was caring, thoughtful, and—in our view—an ideal physician. Unfortunately, by the time he saw Mary, the damage had been done, and his input served only to confirm her final diagnosis. If only our first neurologist had handed Mary's care to this physician or assigned the coordination of her care to a nurse or nurse practitioner, perhaps her entire hospitalization could have been avoided.

Mary's first internist did hand off Mary's care to another physician; however the transfer was rushed. Seamless handoffs that are carefully designed are the hallmark of the Toyota motor vehicle assembly line, and if these handoffs are defective, the quality of the vehicle that is being assembled can be seriously compromised. Football, soccer, volleyball, and basketball players spend hours practicing their handoffs and passes to ensure the receiver does not lose the ball. All coaches preach that effective handoffs and passes spell the difference between victory and defeat.

The principles of manufacturing and athletics also came into play during the first days of Mary's hospitalization. Toyota and other high-performing manufacturers utilize carefully constructed protocols to ensure that each step in the manufacturing process is reliable and stable. Such protocols allow the less experienced members of the assembly line to perform each manufacturing step with nearly the identical skills of a highly experienced employee. Similarly, athletic teams utilize playbooks that carefully define and choreograph the actions of each player and allow each player to more quickly achieve a high level of performance.

In Mary's case, the use of an anticoagulation protocol or playbook would have allowed her inexperienced intern to manage the dosing of her blood thinner (heparin) in the same manner as a highly experienced physician. Alternatively and in most cases, a preferable strategy would have been to allow the bedside nurse to apply the anticoagulation protocol to manage her anticoagulation. Upon entering Mary's blood anticoagulation value into the protocol, the intern or nurse would have been warned that the anticoagulation level was insufficient to prevent further blood clot formation in her leg, and the protocol would have called for an increased infusion rate of her heparin, ensuring administration of a sufficient dose. In the absence of a protocol or empowerment of the bedside nurses to manage the anticoagulation, the intern underdosed Mary's heparin, allowing additional clots to form and migrate from her leg veins into her lungs. These large clots cut off oxygen to her lungs, causing severe damage that resulted in chest pain and shortness of breath.

Who Are the Industry Leaders We Should Emulate?

In order to understand how to mitigate the many lapses in quality observed in Mary's care, everyone who hopes to improve patient care should look to high-performing companies that have risen above their competitors. Although no industry exactly recapitulates the complexities and variables of patient care, many of the practices of these outstanding companies can and should be adapted for patient care. Acknowledging that there are many outstanding companies that could be highlighted, this chapter will focus on leaders from the automotive, airline, and food industries because each of them provides helpful examples of processes those of us in health care need to emulate.

Although Toyota suffered negative publicity in 2010 over the malfunction of an accelerator pedal and a braking system, historically this company has been widely acknowledged as a worldwide leader in the automobile industry. In the past decade, Toyota exceeded the average initial quality ratings of other manufacturers by 20 percent and the average vehicle dependability index

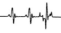

(five-year performance) by 22 percent. Several years ago, an analysis by the Consumers Union revealed that an eight-year-old Toyota was equivalent in reliability to a three-year-old Ford or Chrysler and a two-year-old Volkswagen.

As a consequence of this remarkable performance record, hundreds of books have been written about the Toyota Production System (TPS). Amazon.com lists 204 books on TPS and more than 5,000 books about Toyota. Toyota's competitors have also embraced their production system. As a consequence, the quality of Ford, General Motors, and to a lesser extent, Chrysler, as well as many of the foreign motor vehicle manufacturers, has dramatically improved. Many companies can now rightfully brag that the quality of their cars and trucks is as good as or better than Toyota. The fact remains that Toyota led the way in reducing defects and has devoted more than sixty years to developing a system that fosters continual improvement in quality and reliability. What lessons can health care take away from the Toyota Production System?

Anyone who has flown on Southwest Airlines has witnessed the positive attitude and service orientation of their flight attendants, the efficient passenger seating system, and the time lines of their flights. Southwest won the industry's Triple Crown for the fewest delays, fewest complaints, and fewest mishandled bags for four consecutive years, from 1992–1996, and continues to be one of the leaders in all these categories[1]. Most importantly, Southwest has never experienced an operations-related passenger fatality[2]. What are the secrets to Southwest Airlines' success, and can we in health care learn from it?

For those of you fortunate enough to have a Publix Supermarket in your neighborhood, you have experienced the rich variety of fresh produce; the colorful, well-organized shelf displays; and the squeaky clean floors, combined with friendly, efficient service and highly competitive food prices. This employee-owned supermarket chain has succeeded in an industry where extremely small profit margins and complex supply systems make up the battleground. How does Publix maintain such rigorous operating systems and simultaneously nurture friendly and happy employees who provide exceptional customer service?

Toyota Production System (TPS)

Push Versus Pull Manufacturing

After World War II, Japanese industry was in an extremely sorry state. Estimates of the productivity of the Japanese work force suggested that nine Japanese workers were required to equal the output of one American worker. Toyota admired American productivity and turned to the example of Henry Ford, who continually focused on removing non-value-added waste. Like Henry Ford, Toyota relentlessly pursued the removal of waste to continually improve their "value stream"[3].

However, Toyota realized that modern American manufacturers had forgotten Ford's original example in their quest for ever-greater profits through mass production. Mass production techniques produced large quantities of single models quickly and with lower labor costs; however, these bulk processes created great waste. Furthermore, mass production required American manufacturers to push their products onto the market. The more cars they produced, the greater their need to create demand. Advertising combined with sales promotions was the key to this "push culture." During times of prosperity, this approach generated great profits.

In certain regions of the United States, just like the American automotive industry, physicians have pushed care on their patients by performing unnecessary surgery, ordering unnecessary diagnostic tests, and requiring excessive visits to maximize income. For example the per capita cost of health care in Miami, Florida, was $16,351 in 2006, as compared to Salem, Oregon, at $5,877, and physicians in Miami were far more likely to recommend tests that were not clearly indicated and to schedule unnecessarily frequent office visits[4].

These differences cannot simply be explained away by differences in the cost of living, demographics, or geographic distances. Comparisons of regions within single states and contiguous counties have also uncovered extreme differences in per capita spending on health care. In McAllen, Texas, the per capita cost was second to Miami at $14,946, while in nearby El Paso the health care expenditure averaged $7,504 per person[5]. This statistic is even more shocking when one discovers that the average household income in McAllen was only $12,000. McAllen physicians were motivated by an entrepreneurial spirit and were trained to perform specific procedures. They consistently recommended diagnostic tests or procedures for their patients, disregarding the lack of evidence that these interventions were of benefit. Both doctors and patients assumed that more care was better care. When asked about the high cost of medical care in McAllen, a local surgeon admitted there was "overutilization here, pure and simple"[5].

Analysts agree that a push business philosophy is likely to be one of the primary drivers causing the great variations in per capita health care spending in United States. One of the tenets of capitalism has been, "You get what you pay for." However, patients as well as health care providers need to remember that when it comes to health care, under the present volume-oriented reimbursement system, higher cost health care often translates to more unnecessary procedures and tests. And the more you do, the greater the likelihood of errors and complications.

Analysis of regional health care quality and per capita spending shows no positive correlation. In fact, there may be a subtle negative correlation. In other words, higher cost health care may actually yield worse outcomes than less wasteful, lower cost care[6]. One of the primary charges of the Hippocratic Oath is to "do no harm"[7], and physicians enamored with procedures need to remember this charge (no pun intended) when the indications for a diagnostic or therapeutic procedure are equivocal. When it came to Mary's case, I wonder what benefit her nerve conductions had on her treatment. They seemed to lead the neurologist down the wrong path; they were also expensive, time consuming, and painful.

Toyota subscribes to a "pull" rather than a push approach to car manufacturing; that is, productivity is matched to demand, and the supply of individual parts is determined by starting at the end of the production line, not at the beginning. When a customer asks for a blue Corolla, the order moves backward, requesting a Corolla chassis and engine, as well as the other approximately one thousand parts that make up this automobile. Toyota does not store large inventories of parts, but manufacturers supply each part just in time to meet the demand. What does this approach mean for health care? Health care systems and health care providers need to avoid batch and mass production whenever possible. Furthermore, building excess capacity engenders a push philosophy and over-treatment.

Key Points about Push Versus Pull Manufacturing

- The American automobile industry has utilized mass production, leading to
  - overproduction;
  - increased waste; and
  - lower cost per car.

- Overproduction necessitates that cars be pushed onto the market, which
  - requires advertising and promotions to create new demand and
  - results in high profits during times of prosperity.

- Areas of the country with high numbers of physician specialists
  - often have higher per capita health care costs (Miami, Florida, $16,351 per person) than areas with lower numbers of specialists (Salem, Oregon, $5,877 per person) and
  - do *not* mean higher costs are accompanied by improved health outcomes.

- Toyota uses a pull model that manufactures cars based on customer orders, which leads to
  - minimal waste and
  - potential profits even during economic downturns.

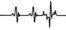

Elimination of Waste

When demand increases, the natural response is to immediately hire more workers and to purchase additional equipment. However, Toyota realized that an organization's productivity could also be greatly increased by aggressively and continually removing waste:

$$Production\ capacity = work - waste$$

By reducing waste, any service or manufacturing organization can increase production capacity without increasing work effort or employee numbers. In health care, increases in patient care demands can also be met by reducing waste, and because nurses are on the front lines, they can be particularly effective at identifying wasteful practices and helping to eliminate them.

There are eight potentially useful approaches to waste reduction[8]:

1. *Don't overproduce.* Many health care providers and hospital systems overproduce and create artificial demand by recommending unnecessary tests and procedures. Doctors that create excess delivery capacity have an inherent conflict of interest in that they both recommend and benefit financially from the procedures and diagnostic tests they perform. When nurses are considering a new position, they should beware of health systems with large new offices and new purchases of equipment because these "improvements" may translate into unneeded tests and procedures for their patients. For example, after a cardiologist practice builds an additional cardiac catheterization laboratory and hires an additional catheterization expert, each patient that comes to their office with chest pain is more likely to undergo this procedure in order to satisfy the excess in cardiac catheterization capacity.

   Medical training programs have produced an excessive number of physicians who perform specific procedures. And these physicians too often push their procedures on unsuspecting patients. Their motto is, "When you have a hammer, everything looks like a nail," and

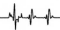

rather than recommending their procedure sparingly for the specific indications approved by the Federal Drug Administration, these physicians often expand their specific procedure to other situations where benefit has not been proven. Nurses can and should speak out about this potentially harmful form of waste.

2. *Use the minimum manpower to achieve your production goals.* In health care we need to continually examine the specific roles of each individual, each team, and each primary care service, as well as supporting services including administration, pharmacy, radiology, laboratory medicine, respiratory care, physical therapy, social service, nutrition support, and housekeeping. Nurses need to continually ask, "Is each person adding true value to my patient's care?" Specific measures of productivity per person and per team need to be utilized to effectively assess patient value. In Mary's case, the number of personnel caring for her was in fact excessive. In all likelihood the large number of health care providers interfered with her care because of the great difficulty in coordinating their input. As will be discussed in Chapter 4, team productivity quickly deteriorates when the team number increases above five or six (see **Figure 4.1** process loss versus personnel number).

3. *Eliminate wasteful time delays.* Delays due to process inefficiencies waste the time of both care providers and patients. Problems of patient flow are a major concern in the health care industry. Anyone who has spent two hours in a waiting room, missing work, lying on a stretcher in the emergency room, waiting for an available hospital bed, or any nurse or physician who has waited for a vacant examining room or an available operating room can attest to the importance of eliminating these delays. In Mary's case, there were serious delays in instituting appropriate therapy as a consequence of an inability to integrate the input of multiple subspecialists.

4. *Eliminate inefficient processes.* In health care there are many processes that have been retained based on past tradition. For example, many residents continue to verbally present complete histories and physicals

the morning after a new patient admission, despite the fact that the dictated admission documents are available in the electronic record. Attending physicians can quickly read these documents before rounds, eliminating the need for such long-winded presentations. During rounds, care providers should be focusing on their new patient's active problems, appropriate diagnostic tests, and timely therapeutic interventions. Most importantly, physicians should be utilizing this valuable time to ensure that care is coordinated and that the bedside nurses understand and participate in formulating the patient's management plans. In Mary's case, there were many lengthy verbal discussions and extensive lists of possible causes of her illness; however, no one integrated her many clinical findings and created an action plan. Nurses were not encouraged to participate on rounds, and their concerns were ignored.

Case 2.1. A middle-aged woman and mother of three was diagnosed with metastatic breast cancer. Her CT scan identified a single metastasis to her lung. She underwent bilateral mastectomies and also had the single lung lesion surgically resected. She then underwent four months of aggressive chemotherapy. She was scheduled for a CT at the end of her chemotherapy and was told that this test would determine whether further therapy would be necessary. She was also apprised that this test would determine whether she could be cured. She waited anxiously for the day of the test, and after the CT was performed in the early morning, she waited to be notified of the results. To her and her family's dismay, no one called that day or the following day. It was not until the third day that her cancer specialist called to inform her that there was no evidence of recurrent tumor and that she was now eligible for adjuvant radiation therapy.

As described in **Case 2.1**, another major inefficiency is the reporting of important diagnostic tests to patients. Imagine being a cancer patient who is waiting for the results of a CT scan to determine if your cancer had responded to chemotherapy. Too often, critical results are not relayed to the patient for several days, creating unnecessary anxiety. Such inefficient processes disrespect our patients, and must be improved.

5. *Avoid large inventories of supplies and equipment.* Space is at a premium in our hospitals and clinics. By avoiding batch processing, large inventories of supplies and equipment are unnecessary. As will be discussed below, a leveling of the workload can eliminate large demand peaks and provide hospitals and clinics with sufficient time to request additional supplies from manufacturers rather than wasting space and money purchasing and storing extra supplies. The supermarket industry has been particularly effective at creating just-in-time supply streams, and the health care industry needs to emulate their successful methods.

6. *Eliminate wasteful movement.* Toyota and many other manufacturers have devoted major efforts to reducing unnecessary human motion, and wasteful equipment and supply movement. In most of our hospitals and clinics, inordinate amounts of time are wasted moving from floor to floor and from room to room. Many inpatient rounding teams are required to see patients on four and five floors, and each change of floor can take up to five minutes.

Inefficiencies in motion are particularly important for bedside nurses. When equipment and supplies are located in distant storage rooms or their patients are in separate, physically distant rooms, nurses waste time moving from place to place (see **Figure 2.5**). When physicians and nurses are required to walk to distant rooms, supply closets, and multiple floors, these wasted motions take away valuable time that could be devoted to direct patient care. Reorganizing processes to reduce movement and transportation requirements promises to greatly enhance the efficiency of many health care systems.

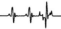

7. *Avoid misdiagnosis and prevent errors.* As Mary's case so dramatically illustrates, misdiagnosis can cause serious harm. The misdiagnosis of the cause of her nerve injury at the beginning of her illness set the diagnostic and therapeutic plans on the wrong trajectory. Her problems were also greatly compounded by errors in the administration of her heparin. What should have been a four-day admission ended up being a nearly month-long hospitalization, requiring expensive equipment and multiple diagnostic studies as well as extensive efforts by highly paid subspecialists, a large team of nurses, and many support staff. The monetary as well as the emotional cost of errors make this category of waste of primary importance.

8. *Harness employee and patient creativity.* Unlike Henry Ford and many of the American car manufacturers who often ignored the needs of their workers, Toyota emphasizes respect for the employees running the machines. They encourage and reward employees who provide suggestions for improvement. Also unlike the American manufacturers who must deal with labor unions and strict work rules that block innovative improvement, Toyota's focus on creating meaningful work and demonstrating respect for all employees has obviated the need for unions. Toyota has emphasized a relatively flat administrative power gradient. Managers are constantly visiting the floors to support those on the assembly line. If medical practices were to follow Toyota's model, the frontline caregivers—particularly nurses, who are actually doing the work of caring for our patients— would be empowered to improve the systems of care. Encouraging greater job autonomy enhances motivation and job satisfaction and reduces employee turnover. By adhering to these approaches, Toyota of North America consistently achieves a job attrition rate of only 2.5 percent[9]. This statistic contrasts starkly with estimated 16–30 percent attrition rates for U.S. nurses[10].

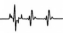
Key Points about Removing Waste
- Removing waste is the most cost effective method for increasing production.

- There are eight ways to reduce waste:
  1. Don't overproduce.
  2. Use the minimum manpower to achieve your goals.
  3. Eliminate time delays.
  4. Eliminate wasteful processes.
  5. Avoid large inventories of supplies and equipment.
  6. Eliminate wasteful movements.
  7. Avoid misdiagnosis and errors.
  8. Harness the creativity of your employees and patients by
     - focusing on employee and patient satisfaction;
     - rewarding suggestions for improvement;
     - encouraging job autonomy; and
     - establishing a flat administrative structure.

In addition to input from nurses, we need to encourage input from patients on how to improve our processes and reduce waste. Being on the receiving end of care provides a useful perspective. Encouraging patient suggestions has the added dividends of improving each patient's sense of control over their care and of improving their satisfaction. Nurses should ask open-ended questions regarding patient satisfaction and relay these comments to administrators. Formal surveys can also be helpful in monitoring overall patient satisfaction.

Work Flow

Another key principle of the Toyota Production System is its emphasis on the steady flow of work[8]. When the flow of work is constant, inventory depletion is predictable and workers are neither idle nor overworked or rushed. These conditions reduce the likelihood of errors and improve quality and job satisfaction. How does Toyota determine appropriate workflow rates? As an

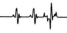

example, let's examine how Toyota calculates the flow rate to manufacture one thousand steering wheels in one month. Achievement of this goal will require that forty steering wheels be produced per day for twenty-five days. A workday has 480 minutes in it; therefore, one steering wheel will need to be manufactured every twelve minutes, and managers will create a specific series of manufacturing protocols to meet this time constraint.

A similar approach should be applied to our hospitals and clinics to improve patient flow. In order to understand the processing of each patient, specific disease value streams need to be constructed (see **Figure 2.1**). One disease that is being carefully monitored by Medicare is pneumonia. One quality measure for pneumonia is the time interval between arrival in the emergency room and the initiation of antibiotic therapy. By defining the key elements of disease management and ensuring rapid and consistent evaluation and testing, this time interval can be reduced to less than one hour, which is three hours below the four-hour limit required by Medicare. Given the fact that most bacteria grow rapidly (doubling in number roughly every sixty minutes), it is easy to see why reducing the time between first encounter and antibiotic treatment is so important.

Pneumonia Value Stream

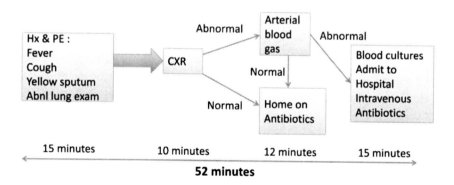

Figure 2.1. Pneumonia value stream. Times for each stage are listed, and the total processing time from arrival in the emergency room to the start of antibiotics can be shortened to less than sixty minutes.

One major impediment to smooth workflow is the large variation in the complexity of the manufacturing processes. In virtually all service and manufacturing organizations, the 80/20 rule applies: 20 percent of the product provides 80 percent of the variation. These more complicated products need to be managed by a "slice and dice" approach (see **Figure 2.2**). A complex product must first be isolated, or sliced, from the standard manufacturing stream and be produced using a separate stream of processing steps. After the creation of a separate flow, planners must break apart, or dice, this new processing stream and focus on improving its most variable and unreliable step. This same approach can be applied to patient care[11]. As in automotive manufacturing, 80 percent of the patients have routine complaints that are readily diagnosed and managed using a predictable sequential approach that can be continually improved.

One excellent example of a highly orchestrated sequential process is cataract surgery. Cataracts are readily diagnosed, and the steps for corrective surgery have been continually improved to the point where surgical time can be reduced to ten minutes[12]. Just as for cataract surgery, teams can be trained to carry out specific pathways that achieve highly reliable sequential care. As these specialty teams gain more experience and continually remove waste, the efficiency, quality, and safety of care will progressively improve.

How should we manage the 20 percent of patients who have complex problems that take up to 80 percent of the health care system's time and resources? For these patients, the diagnosis is often unclear at the time they enter the hospital or arrive in the clinic. Alternatively, there may be insufficient prior scientific and clinical evidence to guide their management, eliminating the possibility of using algorithms. These patients require an iterative approach that progressively decreases diagnostic uncertainty rather than a simple linear sequential approach to care[11]. These patients need to be sliced from the routine medical ward team or primary care clinic and assigned to a team with extensive expertise in iterative problem solving. Ideally such diagnostic teams should consist of the most experienced and talented physicians, nurses, and support staff.

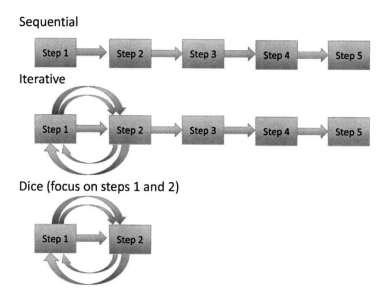

Figure 2.2. Slice and dice. Complex iterative cases should be removed or "sliced" from the usual sequential patient value stream and a second value stream created. The first step of the management of these complex patients should be "diced." That is, the iterative process of narrowing the diagnostic possibilities should be continually analyzed and improved.

Too often, inexperienced physicians and nurse practitioners apply a sequential rather than an iterative approach to complex patients. They may unknowingly activate the wrong sequential pathway, delaying appropriate care and wasting valuable resources. For example, the intern assigned to Mary's case was an ear, nose, and throat (ENT) trainee rotating for one month on the general medicine wards. ENT is a procedure-oriented surgical subspecialty that primarily manages patients with known diagnoses that require predictable sequential care. This intern was unprepared for the complexities of Mary's multisystemic illness. Sadly, to this day, I recall his deer-in-the-headlights expression as Mary's condition deteriorated.

Furthermore, the general medicine internist who initially managed her hospitalization had extensive experience managing chronic diseases such as hypertension and diabetes. To manage these diseases he usually employed well-designed algorithms. Given the predictable nature of his clinical practice, he was ill-prepared to assess the many unusual clinical findings associated with Mary's illness. He and his medical residents suffered from confirmation bias. They assumed that Mary simply had a common disorder—thrombophlebitis. They treated her with standard doses of heparin but failed to manage the sequential process of adjusting her heparin dose.

Eventually realizing that he was incapable of creating a unifying diagnosis, the attending physician consulted multiple specialists; however, he lacked sufficient training and skills to create a true medical team that could integrate the input of the consultants. To make conditions even more difficult, Mary was hospitalized within a population of far simpler sequential patients, and this arrangement prevented her physicians and nurses from fully appreciating the complexity and dangerous nature of her illness.

Not only is it important to segregate sequentially managed patients from iteratively managed patients to improve care and patient flow, but it is also important to establish separate reimbursement models[13]. Patients receiving specific value-added services that require sequential care, such as a cataract surgery, kidney transplant, cardiac catheterization, or pacemaker placement, should be charged a predetermined fixed fee for each of these value-added services. This fee structure would allow patients to shop for the hospital or clinic with the best price. Sequential services also lend themselves well to determining quality measures, such as measuring postoperative complications, length of stay, and readmission rates. These measures, when publicly shared, would allow potential customers to make decisions based on quality in addition to price. From the standpoint of the care delivery teams, the setting of specific prices would encourage continual reductions in waste because improvements in efficiency would be expected to reduce cost and improve net earnings.

In recognition of the inability to predict expenses for patients requiring iterative management, the billing structure should be based on an hourly rate until a diagnosis is secured. At that juncture, a sequential care billing system could be activated. Initially, insurance companies are likely to be uncomfortable with this arrangement; however, at the present time the reimbursement of sequentially managed patients is cross-subsidizing these more complex and resource-intensive iterative patients.

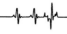

By creating two separate value streams and two separate business models, patient flow and efficiency could be improved, bringing down costs while simultaneously improving the quality of care[13]. In today's reimbursement system, many entrepreneurs have focused on "skimming the cream" by creating highly profitable specialty hospitals that admit only patients requiring sequential care. These hospitals triage patients who must receive expensive and poorly reimbursed iterative care to general hospitals and university medical centers, contributing to the poor financial state of many of those institutions.

> **Case 2.2.** Ms. Jones was admitted to the hospital because of fever and severe shaking chills following dialysis. Her blood cultures grew *Staphylococcal aureus* that was resistant to the antibiotic methicillin (also called MRSA). Because she developed hypotension and appeared very ill, her dialysis catheter had to be removed, and she was treated with the intravenous antibiotic vancomycin. She rapidly improved. On Friday she was scheduled to have her dialysis catheter reinserted by the X-ray department and discharged home. Upon arrival at the catheter placement suite at 2:00 p.m., she discovered her procedure had been canceled because she had been skipped over (bumped) for an emergency catheter placement. The radiologist informed her that she would have to remain in the hospital until Monday because he was leaving at 2:00 p.m. and didn't work on the weekend. Ms. Jones began crying. Both her nurse and the ward physician called the X-ray department and pleaded but to no avail. Ms. Jones had to wait in the hospital for two extra days before she could receive her catheter on Monday.

Other Impediments to Efficient Patient Flow

Hospitalized patients require services from multiple departments, and all too often one or more of the services fails to fulfill its obligation to the patient. The consequences are blocks in patient flow and the unnecessary prolongation of hospital stays. In **Case 2.2**, both the nurse and internist caring for Ms. Jones were in different departments than the radiologist, and they had no authority to insist that the catheter be placed in a timely fashion. The radiologist did not respect the needs of either the patient or her caregivers but rather focused on his own desire to leave the hospital. This all too common occurrence exemplifies the problems with department silos and poor customer-supplier relationships. Effective administrative structures break down silos. For example, each patient could be assigned a care coordinator or operations manager who is empowered to override individual caregivers who ignore the needs of the patients and obstruct patient flow.

Case 2.3. Mrs. Williams had worked for many years as an office clerk. Her pay was modest, and she received no health insurance benefits. Her husband was a self-employed carpenter who also made a modest living. They had raised five fully-grown and productive children and for years had expended a significant percentage of their income to buy health insurance. The highlight of each summer was their vacation in the Blue Ridge Mountains, but eventually because of the increases in their health insurance premiums, they were forced to choose between health insurance coverage and their beloved annual Blue Ridge Mountain vacation.

Mrs. Williams chose to discontinue her insurance. The next time she visited her primary care physician, she informed him that she could not fully pay him for her visit. He became upset, and she felt ashamed. She never sought his care again. A year later she developed painful redness on her abdomen. She applied hot soaks to the area, but the redness continued to expand. She remained at home despite her worsening pain and the onset of fever and chills. When she lost consciousness, her husband rushed her to the emergency room, where the diagnosis of a flesh eating Group A Streptococcal infection was made, and she underwent extensive surgical resection of the irreversibly damaged abdominal tissue. She was admitted to the intensive care unit, where she died. Her son observed tearfully, "My mom is dead because she loved the Blue Ridge Mountains."

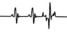

GATEWAY

ENTER

TWO

http://bit.ly/vCh0WT

Key Points about Work Flow

- A constant and steady work flow increases efficiency and quality.
  - ○ Requires planning to create predictable flow
  - ○ Total product or service units/total time = time per unit

- Adapt flow to take into account the 80/20 rule.
  - ○ Health care systems need to "slice and dice" (i.e., separate) complex iterative patients from sequential patients and focus on their diagnosis.
  - ○ Iterative patients
    - ▪ require highly experienced personnel and
    - ▪ should have a per-hour billing structure.
  - ○ Sequential patients
    - ▪ can be managed by algorithms and
    - ▪ should have a fixed price billing structure.

- Create administrative structures that eliminate obstructions to flow.
  - ○ Department silos impair customer-supplier relationships.
  - ○ An operations manager is required to supervise individual patient flow.

- Reduce emergency room admissions because they
  - ○ lead to unpredictable peaks and flows and
  - ○ reflect poor access to primary care.

Another major impediment to stable and smooth workflow in many hospitals is the high number of emergency room admissions. These patients are unscheduled, making proper personnel and hospital bed allocations impossible. This condition requires that hospitals maintain an excess bed capacity and a buffer of extra employees stationed in the hospital. As in **Case 2.3**, many emergency room admissions represent a failure of the health care system. When patients lack access to health care providers, they live with their medical complaints until their symptoms become intolerable, and then they are forced to seek care in the emergency room.

Sudden arrivals of sick patients can quickly overtax inpatient medical teams, resulting in patient management errors. Ideally each patient should have a primary care provider who assesses and treats their complaints before they become extreme and who—when a more serious therapeutic intervention is required—can schedule a hospital admission. In Mrs. Williams's case, the primary care provider could have ordered an oral antibiotic and then scheduled admission to the hospital if her abdominal infection failed to respond. This approach would have resulted in a more predictable hospital admission, allowed the creation of a smoother workflow, and saved Mrs. Williams's life.

Creating Conditions that Reduce Waste and Improve Flow

In order to ensure waste reduction and smooth production flow, Toyota and other high-performing manufacturers and service industries establish three critical conditions for all work[14].

1. *The creation of standard work sheets and protocols*—Carefully designed protocols allow inexperienced workers to function at the level of an expert. Employees in these organizations understand that protocols are created to set the stage for further improvement. If job descriptions are ambiguous and each process is randomly performed, when an error or waste is identified, these conditions cannot be improved because there is no fixed operating process to modify. When workers first learn through simulation and then utilize carefully designed protocols on the front lines, they learn by doing and eventually

develop highly effective habits that can be managed subconsciously. When routines become background activities, each worker's mental activity can focus on the characteristics of their service or product that don't match with their usual experience. The ability to quickly identify the abnormal allows those on the front lines to correct errors rapidly. As discussed earlier, if a protocol had been in place to guide Mary's heparin therapy, she would never have suffered a pulmonary embolus. Furthermore, the use of a protocol that becomes habitual frees mental energy to design improvements in each work process.

2. *Stable and well-defined customer-supplier relationships*—At Toyota, each assembly worker understands that the next worker in the assembly line is his or her customer. Their job is to supply that downstream worker with a perfect product. And the entire workforce is dedicated to never allowing a defect or error to reach the customer. In health care, many of the customer-supplier relationships are poorly understood, and these dysfunctional relationships account for many of the preventable errors suffered by our patients. There is a series of important customer-supplier relationships that need to be stable and well defined, including physician-nurse, physician-patient, nurse-patient, and physician-physician relationships.

Many physicians fail to realize that when they order medications, their primary customers are the bedside nurses responsible for administering the treatments. Too often physicians incorrectly regard nurses as their suppliers. In the steep hierarchies of many medical cultures, including the one where Mary was cared for, nurses are expected to be deferential to physicians and to automatically follow their orders. However, too often the instructions provided by physicians are ambiguous, which increases the likelihood of an error.

When nurses feel they must be suppliers of physician ego gratification, they are less likely to question unclear or incorrect physician orders. When this customer-supplier relationship is dysfunctional, nurses may feel obligated to make an educated guess as to the meaning of an order and supply a medication to the patient despite concerns about the dose or the effectiveness of the medication. These assumptions increase the likelihood of a harmful error that will not only to hurt the patient but also cause emotional harm to the well-meaning nurse. In Mary's case, the nurses were fearful of speaking up and correcting her heparin dose.

Case 2.2 illustrates dysfunctional physician-patient, physician-nurse, and physician-physician customer supplier relationships. The radiologist scheduled to place Ms. Jones's intravenous dialysis catheter did not regard the patient, the bedside nurse, or internal medicine physician as his customers. Imagine if a salesperson at Best Buy refused to sell you an expensive television set because he or she wanted to leave early. Would you ever return to that store again? How long do you think that salesperson would have a job? Sadly, in many cases patients feel they are captives in their health care systems, and too often they fail to realize the dysfunctional nature of those who are supposed to be supplying their care. In Mary's case, I accepted the fact that the neurologist had left for a conference without coverage and worked around the problem by taking her to see a general internist. Similarly, nurses and physicians accept these dysfunctional relationships as simply "the way it is." Patients need to understand that they are the ultimate customers, and both nurses and physicians need to respect this most important relationship.

When a fellow caregiver is ignoring this central relationship, nurses and physicians need to strongly advocate for their patients. One of the most effective ways of overriding delays is to say, "Our patient is depending on you for his/her care. Won't you help me to provide the best possible care for our patient?" Many health care systems are now emphasizing patient-centered care. If this goal has been espoused by your medical center, those of you who are bedside nurses should devote your energies to ensuring that your institution is living up its promise by insisting your patients be treated as esteemed and valued customers.

Another important customer-supplier relationship is established when a caregiver hands off the care of his/her patients to another

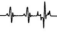

caregiver[15]. Nurses are required to sign out their patients at the end of each shift. The goal of the nurse going off duty is to reliably and accurately transfer information about each patient to the nurse who is taking over the responsibility for care.

In some hospitals, floors nurses transfer or discharge 40–70 percent of their patients every day. Recently nurses have begun transferring information about their patients at the bedside to ensure that they hand off the most current information and involve each patient in the transfer of nursing care.

Best practices for transferring patient care are continuing to evolve. Many hospitals are embracing the use of SBAR:

- *situation* (What significant medical events occurred during your shift?)

- *background* (Why was the patient admitted and what has happened since admission?)

- *assessment* (What do you think is going on?)

- *recommendations* (What diagnostic and therapeutic interventions do you feel should be implemented?).

SBAR is efficient and ensures significant factual content[16, 17].

The bedside handoff should also include verbal acknowledgements of key facts and active questioning by the recipient and be accompanied by a typewritten or electronically generated sign-out to ensure retention of the highest factual content. Computerized sign-out sheets can provide accurate and detailed information on each patient and eliminate the need to spend valuable time copying and collating patient data[18]. And handheld electronic devices promise to improve the portability of these programs[19].

3. *A commitment to continual improvement*—Employees and patients should feel empowered to suggest improvements in efficiency. To accomplish this goal, everyone should be familiar with the scientific

method. They must learn how to generate a hypothesis and test it. Toyota trains their workers to carry out repeated improvement cycles consisting of *plan, do, check, act* (PDCA):

- Plan—Develop an action plan to improve a process.

- Do—Try to implement the new plan.

- Check—Ensure that your plan had the intended results.

- Act—Make adjustments to your original plan based on your check, and repeat the cycle again.

Through repeated cycles of PDCA and under the guidance of expert coaching, each manufacturing process can be continually improved. This same approach has been effectively used to reduce errors and improve quality in health care, which will be discussed in more detail in the next chapter.

Case 2.4. Nurses on an active medical floor were assigned the responsibility of monitoring the infection isolation carts to ensure they were stocked with isolation gowns, gloves, and masks. Several times per day, one or two of the carts ran out of gowns. Rather than notifying the supply manager, the nurses chose to run down to the supply room at the end of the hall and restock the carts—a job that was not assigned to them. Calculations revealed that on average each nurse expended fifteen minutes per day restocking the isolation carts.

Too often those on the front lines assume that all improvements require high-level administrative intervention, and as a consequence they fail to take charge of the many changes they can readily bring about. As shown in **Figure 2.3**, the majority of organizational process improvements are small and do not require high-level administrative input. As described in **Case 2.4**, providers on the front lines experience these smaller process defects daily. Because there are no administrative pathways to improve these small steps, workers are encouraged to create work-around solutions. Recognizing that work-around solutions are wasteful, Toyota employees are encouraged and empowered to permanently eliminate all wasteful processes. These activities involve active discussions with fellow employees and supervisors. In many instances work teams are assembled. Once the team has agreed upon a solution, they pilot the improvement. When finally perfected by multiple PDCA cycles, the new practice is then disseminated throughout the factory.

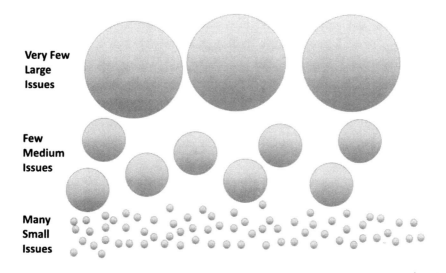

Figure 2.3. Typical relative numbers of improvement opportunities. The majority of problems are small and can be managed by those on the front lines without the need for higher-level administration. A few issues need middle management input, and only a few large system-wide problems require the input of high-level administrators[8]

How can health care systems administrators encourage continual improvement on the frontlines? One potential solution is to adopt a unit-based leadership model consisting of a physician leader, a nurse leader, and a quality coordinator who together take on frontline administrative responsibility for a defined area of a hospital or clinic[20]. These local administrators can involve caregivers and patients in improving each unit's value stream. The quality coordinator can use patient surveys, length of stay, and readmission data to provide performance feedback to the patient care team. By holding a weekly operational meeting, all roadblocks to care can be discussed, and frontline caregivers can be empowered to suggest and pilot improvements. This administrative model promises to build a learn-by-doing culture (see below) that embraces continuous waste reduction and quality improvement.

If the nurses in **Case 2.4** had used Toyota's approach, they would have notified the appropriate administrator and formed a work team to create a permanent solution to their problem. By creating a resupply protocol that increased the involvement of the support staff responsible for supplies, they could have permanently eliminated this distracting task. A unit leadership structure could have facilitated these activities by establishing a more transparent administrative structure and a clear customer-supplier relationship (administration supplying the nurses by restocking the isolation carts). A permanent solution would have allowed each nurse to devote fifteen additional minutes to the care of his or her patients. Many unschooled in the culture of continual waste reduction will regard a fifteen-minute reduction as trivial; however, multiple small improvements, each eliminating five to fifteen minutes of unnecessary work, have the potential to remove hours of wasted effort. Multiple small steps can eventually add up to a very large upward step in efficiency.

Finally, the negative publicity Toyota received in 2010 provides a key lesson on the importance of transparency with regard to errors. Toyota has a policy of never letting errors reach the customer. When an assembly worker observes a defect, he or she pulls a cord that sets off an alarm, notifying the team leader to come immediately to the site where the defect was discovered. The team supervisor quickly determines the underlying cause of the defect and, with help of his assembly team, makes a correction that prevents further defects. If a corrective action cannot be established within a short period, the entire assembly line is shut down.

However, Toyota had no such system to identify and correct defects once their cars had left the factory. Consequently, when customers first reported accelerator and brake defects, there were delays in notifying other customers and correcting these defects. These delays endangered customers and dealt a severe blow to Toyota's reputation for quality. Similarly, the institution and physicians who cared for Mary never acknowledged their errors to the public or to me. This generated distrust on my part and motivated me to write publically about

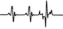

my experiences. When errors occur in manufacturing or in health care, they must be openly discussed and shared with customers or trust and reputation can quickly be destroyed.

Key Points about How to Set Conditions that Encourage Waste Reduction and Improve Flow

1. Create standard work sheets and protocols.
   - Establishes a platform or stage for further improvement
   - Allows inexperienced employees to function at a higher level
   - Allows frontline employees to improve each process

2. Establish stable and reliable customer-supplier relationships.
   - Nurse should be the customer, and the physician the supplier of clear and accurate orders.
   - Nurses signing out their patients are the suppliers of accurate and clear information to the nurse taking over care.

3. Empower all employees to continually improve the processes of care.
   - Teach and practice a scientific approach to problem solving.
   - Plan-do-check-act (PDCA) cycles
   - Avoid work-around solutions by establishing a local, unit-based administrative structure.
   - Remember, many small improvement steps can add up to a major advance.

Southwest Airlines

Southwest began as a small local airline headquartered in Love Field, Texas. The goal of the founding CEO, Herb Kelleher, was to compete with automobiles and buses for short distance transportation. He chose to fly to smaller airports with reduced airline traffic and created a point-to-point rather than a hub-and-spoke network.

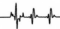

His business model was considered heretical because in the airline industry, long flights generated more profit than more labor intensive short flights, and a hub-and-spoke network model was estimated to generate 20 percent greater revenue than a point-to-point network[1]. In addition, Southwest consistently paid salaries that were comparable to the major airlines. Furthermore, they hired more employees per flight than other airlines, hiring one operations coordinator per flight rather than the industry average of one per three flights and one supervisor per twelve gate employees versus the industry average of one per forty.

These choices eliminated reductions in labor cost as an avenue for improved net revenue. Despite all of these potential impediments, Southwest has steadily grown at rates of 10–15 percent per year for thirty-eight years, and based on the number of scheduled flights, it is now the second largest airline in the world.

How has Southwest overcome the potential obstacles of its business model and achieved such remarkable success? Unlike virtually all its competitors, Southwest has been able to simultaneously improve efficiency and improve quality. Many companies, in their attempt to improve efficiency, cut employees and make everyone work faster. Too often the consequence is reduced quality. However, just as can be observed at Toyota, Southwest has effectively removed waste by eliminating processes that add no value. Rather than depending on someone who is sitting in a distant office on a computer to coordinate the servicing of each airplane as it lands, Southwest assigns one operating agent to work at each gate. The operating agent's primary role is to coordinate the eleven physically separated functional groups that prepare the plane for takeoff:

1. Pilots
2. Flight attendants
3. Gate agents
4. Ticketing agents
5. Ramp agents
6. Baggage transfer agents
7. Cargo agents

8. Mechanics
9. Fuelers
10. Aircraft cleaners
11. Caterers

Whenever possible, the operations agent communicates face-to-face and troubleshoots to ensure that each functional group arrives at the right place at the right time. This masterful coordination results in an average plane turnaround time of twenty to thirty minutes, far below the average of the other airlines, which is twice as long, averaging fifty-five minutes. By eliminating wasted time, Southwest is able to keep its planes—their most valuable asset—in the air for higher percentage of the time as compared to other airlines[1].

To further improve the coordination of these many functional groups, Southwest has a higher proportion of supervisors to employees: one supervisor to twelve employees. The supervisor works alongside his or her employees when there is a shortage of labor. By working on the front lines with supervisees, he or she gains their confidence, builds trust, and flattens the sense of hierarchy. In addition to filling in with extra labor, the supervisor coaches, mentors, co-ordinates, problem-solves, and troubleshoots. Southwest's emphasis on mutual respect also enhances teamwork. Unlike some airlines where the pilots are arrogant and self-righteous, and where airline hostesses disrespect ramp agents, Southwest employees encourage and practice mutual respect. Their code of behavior strongly discourages offending another employee. Employees understand that every job in their team is critical, and this attitude fosters teamwork[1]. Physicians also need to practice mutual respect. Arrogant physicians increase the sense of hierarchy and interfere with teamwork, just like arrogant pilots. In a Southwest culture, physicians would understand that they are part of a team and that they need to work alongside, not over, other health care providers.

Just as coordination of functional groups charged with preparing a plane for takeoff can shorten a plane's turnaround time, the coordination of the many geographically dispersed functional groups responsible for each patient's care could dramatically reduce the time each patient is required to remain in the hospital. The hospital is the system's most valuable asset, and

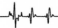

improving patient turnaround time has the potential to substantially increase the number of patients cared for each day.

One of the missing positions in most health care systems is a patient operations agent or care coordinator, someone who could span the many departments that are supposed to work together to provide each patient's care. Many hospital floors have a case manager and/or a social worker; however, their primary task is usually discharge planning. In most systems, no single employee has the sole responsibility for coordinating the many complex steps required to diagnose and treat each hospitalized patient. Imagine if there had been such a coordinator for Mary's hospitalization. That person could have integrated the input of the many consultants and the myriad of laboratory findings, and a clear compilation of all these findings and suggestions would have greatly facilitated the experienced internal medicine attending physician in arriving at an appropriate diagnosis.

How can health care systems create a supervisory structure that is as effective as Southwest's? The unit-based leadership structure described previously could serve this supervisory role. Just like the Southwest supervisors, the physician and nurse unit leaders could work alongside their clinical care teams to increase trust and encourage communication. These leaders could also serve as coaches and mentors, as well as assist in eliminating administrative roadblocks to care.

Southwest also improves efficiency by embracing simplicity. They have one type of aircraft, the Boeing 737, which has a standardized cockpit. This minimizes the training requirements for the pilots, mechanics, cleaners, and other employees and reduces the risk of errors. They also have an open seating system policy that encourages passengers to check in early and arrive early to the airport. This system also eliminates the need for complex and expensive computer reservation algorithms. Finally, they serve no in-flight meals, reducing the caterer's loading time and reducing food storage space.

Caregivers need to follow Southwest's example and continually try to simplify every process. Common floor layouts and common equipment designs can reduce the need for reorientation of nurses when they work in different parts of the hospital or clinic. A single model of each instrument type reduces

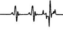

the need for continual retraining to operate different intravenous pumps and cardiac monitoring systems. Simplification not only saves time and money but also improves safety. As will be discussed in the next chapter, the more steps in any procedure and the more complex and varied the equipment, the higher the probability of an error.

Key Points about How to Enhance Coordination and Simplicity

- Assign an operations coordinator to span multiple distant service sites and
  - utilize face-to-face meetings to assure coordination;
  - troubleshoot as necessary; and
  - serve as the interpersonal glue and maintain focus on the care of the patient.

- Create a unit-based supervisory structure where a physician and nurse leader will
  - work side by side with the care team;
  - troubleshoot; and
  - mentor.

- Simplify all processes by removing steps, using common floor layouts, and using common equipment.

Publix Supermarkets

George Jenkins, the founder of Publix supermarkets, started in the grocery business at age seventeen, working for the Florida grocery store chain called Piggly Wiggly. After an Atlanta firm purchased the chain, Mr. George, as he was fondly called, noticed that the new owners never visited his store. Frustrated, he traveled to Atlanta to meet with his new boss, but upon arrival he was told that the boss did not have time to meet with him. As he sat in the waiting area, he overheard his new boss going on and on about his golf game. The next day, Mr. George resigned and invested his life savings to open the first Publix grocery store in Winter Haven, Florida.

At the inception of the company in 1930, all grocers hand-carried the food ordered by the customer to the front counter. Customer service was central to the food business at that time, and customers raved about Publix's friendly service. However, in less than a decade the first self-service grocery stores began to open. Mr. George, fearful of losing the person-to-person contact that had made his store so successful initially, resisted this change, but in 1940 he opened Publix's first self-service food market. To please his customers he added a number of extras, including a dedicated parking lot (most food stores only had parking on the street), air conditioning, a water fountain, and an electric door that automatically opened for the customers as they carried their groceries to their cars.

Case 2.5. An elderly Publix customer rushed into the store, carrying a beautifully decorated birthday cake. As she walked through the door, she was crying uncontrollably. The store manager quickly took her to the employee lounge to calm her down and to find out what was troubling her. He learned that the birthday cake was for her ten-year-old granddaughter who had terminal leukemia. This would be her last birthday, and everything had to be perfect. She had ordered her granddaughter's favorite pound cake, but the bakery had accidently used lemon cake. The birthday party was at 7:30 p.m., and it was now 6:00 p.m. The bakers had left for the day, but the manager and clerk sprung into action. They found four pound cakes but needed six. The manager sent the store clerk to a nearby Publix branch to find two more. Upon the clerk's return, the manager—who had previously worked as a mason—carefully assembled the cakes and smoothly applied the icing, and the clerk placed the trim and the decorations. They found a cashier who had beautiful handwriting to script the birthday greeting. The manager quickly drove the cake to the birthday house, delivering it with ten minutes to spare. Everyone was delighted. The grandmother was still crying. Four weeks later, she returned, again in tears. Her granddaughter had died. The manager and store clerk also cried as they comforted her[21].

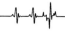
To encourage a continual focus on the customer, Mr. George hired employees who were outgoing, courteous, and helpful and who showed initiative. He always encouraged extra effort and extra service, and he ended every orientation by stating, "If there is ever a customer you can't handle, give them my phone number, because I will." As exemplified in **Case 2.5**, he expected everyone to possess the desire to reach out to the customer, and he sought employees who truly wanted to serve their customers. He realized from the very beginning that the secret to Publix's success was people. To memorialize and reinforce this important principle, he placed this reminder in every store: Publix will be a little better place, or not quite as good... because of you[21]. He believed and modeled exceptional service and wanted his employees to regard exceptional service as the expected norm.

In 1949, he created the Publix slogan: Where Shopping is a Pleasure. His goal was for everyone to enjoy shopping in Publix[21]. He wanted all his employees and his company to be honest and reliable, and these goals were reflected in the company's guarantee:

> Publix guarantees that we will never knowingly disappoint you. If for any reason your purchase does not give you complete satisfaction, the full purchase price will be cheerfully refunded immediately upon request. We have always believed that no sale is complete until the meal is eaten and enjoyed[23].

Shouldn't our health care system have a similar continual focus on pleasing and comforting our patients? All health care providers need to guarantee that we will not disappoint our patients by forcing them to wait for prolonged periods, by failing to explain the plans for their care, and by not being emotionally available to comfort them in times of need.

I am quite sure that Mr. George would never have hired the physicians who first cared for Mary. The final sentence in the Publix guarantee is particularly important regarding Mary's care and the care of all patients. The caregiver's obligation should not end when the patient walks out the door. If for any reason a patient's health is not truly improved by a caregiver's service,

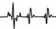

that person should feel obligated to make things right. Patients should expect a "Publix guarantee" from their caregivers. They should expect the same exceptional service that customers receive at this remarkable supermarket. After all, they are not simply purchasing food; they are purchasing an even more fundamental product: their health and well-being.

How does Publix reward and promote its culture of exceptional service? Recognizing that people were his most important asset, Mr. George made all his employees associates of his business. He gave each associate a personal stake by contributing 9–11 percent of their monthly salary to purchase stock in the company. Publix stock has never been available to the public, and it can only be purchased as an employee.

If a Publix associate had purchased $100 of stock in 1959 (the start date of their current stock option plan), those same shares would have been worth $138,802 in May of 2004. Ownership established a unique dynamic in the company because each manager supervised associates who were co-owners, establishing a customer-supplier relationship that reduced the gradient of power and increased trust as well as bi-directional accountability.

Secondly, all customer letters complimenting employees were publically posted, and service awards were given to recognize exceptional service. But most importantly, Mr. George realized that placing the needs of others before self provided its own powerful reward. He also understood that people naturally wanted to identify with not only an organization that was successful but also one that was genuinely good.

Because most hospitals and health systems are presently nonprofit and because co-ownership by health care providers would create serious conflicts of interest, stock options are not a viable reward system for health care providers. However, a strong identification with a "good" health care organization and rewards that encourage, recognize, and sustain outstanding service to patients have the potential to improve how health care providers deliver care. In previous decades, nurses and physicians commonly went beyond the expected, and our professions expected this behavior. However,

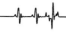

with the institution of new work rules and a change in generational norms, such behavior is now rare. Those of us in health care need to keep in mind the inspirational example of Mr. George and once again make exceptional service the expected.

So how successful is Publix? From its humble beginnings of one store in Winter Haven, Florida, the company has expanded to 1,023 retail locations in five states—Florida, Georgia, South Carolina, Tennessee, and Alabama—and now employs 140,500 people. Publix has been rated by Fortune Magazine as one of the top ten best companies to work for (2005–2008) and is one of Forbes Magazine's top ten largest private companies (2009). Publix consistently scores higher than any other supermarket for customer satisfaction based on the national American Customer Satisfaction Index survey (1995–2010).

Key Points about Customer Service

- Health care providers need to continually focus on serving their patients.

- All health care systems need to emphasize to their employees that the hospital or clinic *"...will be a little better place, or not quite as good...because of you."*

- Institutions must reward exceptional customer service.

- Placing the needs of others before self provides a powerful internal reward.

- A patient satisfaction guarantee could encourage commitment to patients after they walk out the door of the hospital or the clinic.

- Going above and beyond should not be the exception but the norm.

Conclusions about Industry and Health Care

Publix's culture of exceptional customer service, combined with the promotion of systems and teamwork by Toyota and Southwest Airlines, can lead to remarkable competitive advantages. If only our health care providers could emulate the remarkable successes of Toyota, Southwest and Publix, we could all happily live to be one hundred years old!

We All Understand Team Sports

Industry provides wonderful examples for health care providers to emulate; however, many in the medical professions protest that patients are not cars, airplanes, or groceries. Furthermore, most caregivers have little formal business experience and are unfamiliar with manufacturing systems and customer-supplier relationships. A value stream to them sounds like a great place to catch tasty trout.

On the other hand, nearly everyone throughout the world watches and/or has played a team sport. In South and Central America, as well as in Europe and parts of Asia, football (called soccer in the United States) has a passionate following. The World Cup football series is the most watched of all sporting events. To succeed at the highest level, players must practice reciprocal interdependence. They change their positions in response to the movements of their teammates and the opposition. There is constant communication, and the ball is passed to different players on the team, seeking the unguarded player who can kick the ball into the goal. Just like the airline gate support staff at Southwest Airlines, everyone must understand their roles and coordinate their actions to successfully score a goal. And just like workers at Toyota, they follow specific plays or protocols to successfully and efficiently pass the ball from player to player in order to create the opportunities to score.

University of Florida Championship Athletics

Over the past decade, the University of Florida has excelled in its athletic endeavors, and I describe these teams in detail not because I am a fanatic fan or believe that this university has a monopoly on athletic excellence, but rather I describe these teams because I have close personal knowledge of the coaches, the players, and the teams. The women's volleyball team has won the Southeastern Conference Championship eighteen out of the last nineteen years, has reached the final four at the nationals six times, and has reached NCAA finals once over this same time period, and was ranked number one in the nation for much of the 2010 season. The football team (American football) has won three national championships (1996, 2006, and 2008) and has been consistently ranked among the top twenty NCAA Division I-A college football teams in the nation for over a decade.

As the opposition enters the University of Florida (UF) stadium, fans scream "Gator bait!" as they clap in unison with their arms extended, mimicking the chomping motion of alligator jaws. Following each team's seemingly inevitable victory, they chant, "It's great to be a Florida Gator." In addition to the great joy these many victories bring to fans, these remarkable athletic teams provide important lessons for how to improve health care. And the application of these championship athletic principles can begin to transform the nation's health care delivery system into one of which the University of Florida coaches could be proud.

The University of Florida Women's Volleyball Team

As Mary Wise, the women's volleyball coach, stands on the edge of the sidelines, she closely watches her players' every move. Her assistant coaches signal specific plays in response to the tactics of the opposing team. Her team strategy may quickly change depending on the success of her players. Tonight against Auburn, the team is cruising. The UF setter, Chanel Brown, carefully pops the volleyball up near the right side of the net, allowing All-American Kelly Murphy to leap into the air, quickly stretch her right arm behind her head, and hammer the ball across the net with such force and speed that the opposing players don't even have time to flinch. The ball whizzes by, landing inbounds. Kelly has scored her tenth kill.

By the time the match ended, Florida had won three sets to Auburn's zero. Kelly accumulated a total of fifteen kills, while Kristy Jaeckel contributed nine, Callie Rivers had six, Lauren Bledsoe had five, and both Cassandra Anderson and Tangerine Wiggs had four. In the first set, the team succeeded in 37 percent of their kill attempts, as compared to only 6.5 percent for Auburn. During the match, players continually huddled as they patted each other on the back and often shared high fives. When a player made an error, the other players simply nodded encouragement, as if to say, "That's okay, we'll get the next point." The mutual support and admiration within team was apparent to all. Coach Wise was pleased with their outstanding team effort[22].

One of the most important practices nursing administrators need to emulate is Mary Wise's steadfast physical presence close to her players. To understand and support the minute-to-minute needs of our patients on the hospital wards and in the clinics, those in charge must be present on the front lines. Spending the majority of time in distant offices does not consistently add value to our patients' care, and frontline management should be the rule, not the exception.

The high success percentage of Coach Wise's players reflects their mastery of the fundamentals of passing, positioning, and hitting. The efficient motion of Chanel Brown as she set up the kill and the powerful swing of Kelly Murphy demonstrated no wasted motion. By reducing the time between the set and the kill, they gave the opposing players no time to set up a blocking defense, increasing the likelihood of a successful kill. To achieve these outcomes, the volleyball team practices on average three hours a day, and much of that time is devoted to hitting technique, jumping, blocking, and moving quickly into the proper position on the court. Each practice is carefully scheduled several hours before its start to ensure that every minute is effectively devoted to improving the players' and the team's performance.

Similarly, health care providers need to devote greater attention and effort to the fundamentals of communication, coordination, rounding, documentation, and ordering. If health care providers could adhere to predetermined schedules, both on the inpatient service and in the outpatient clinics, patient waiting times and the lengths of hospital stays could be reduced.

Just as these athletes learn the fundamentals of volleyball by practicing proper technique over and over again, caregivers can best learn how to improve their fundamentals by continual supervised practice. Experience has shown that lectures and verbal instruction fail to reliably alter dysfunctional processes. Consistent long-term improvement can only be achieved by repetition under the guidance of frontline coaches. Just like athletes, nurses must learn by doing. Practice can take place on the wards and in the clinics under game conditions with real patients. However, ideally these fundamentals should first be taught by simulation exercises. Simulation should be repeated until the trainee demonstrates consistency and reliability. In the past few years, coaches in many sports have turned to computer simulation to improve athletic performance, and those in health care should emulate this strategy.

Finally, Coach Wise has recognized that women seek to bond with their teammates and achieve victory as a team. Unlike men, who often jockey for supremacy, encourage a hierarchy, and value independence, women prefer to create a web of relationships and a more horizontal group structure. While winning is most important to men, women value attachment and team chemistry. Women athletes love competition, but they prefer competition in the context of a true team[23]. A networking model that encourages identification with the team rather than focusing on individual needs is the ideal approach for achieving highly functional teams in business and in health care, and our health care teams should emulate the example of the highly successful University of Florida women's volleyball team.

GATEWAY

http://bit.ly/s98lau

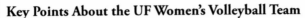
> **Key Points About the UF Women's Volleyball Team**
> - Coaches and administrators need to manage from the front lines.
>
> - The fundamentals of communication and coordination must first be mastered before any system can be mastered.
>
> - Time management is critical, and when possible, schedules should predetermined for all processes and procedures.
>
> - Everyone learns best by
>   - simulation and progress toward real game conditions.
>   - continual coaching.
>
> - Leaders encourage team members to create a supportive network or web and focus on performing and winning as a team.

The University of Florida Football Team

The University of Florida football team met the University of Oklahoma team for the BCS National Championship game in January of 2009. The game was low scoring and close. The first quarter was scoreless, and at half time the teams were tied at 7-7. At the beginning of the fourth quarter, Oklahoma passed for a touchdown, and the score was again tied at 14. The momentum had shifted to Oklahoma. Florida started the next offensive series at its own 22 yard line. Their offensive coordinator, Steve Addazio, called for a trap play— one of the most difficult but potentially one of the most effective running plays in football. The trap play was one of the highest-risk (because of potential errors and fumbles) but highest-gain (could create a very large gap in the defensive line) plays he had in his offensive armamentarium.

Coach Addazio knew they needed a big play. It was now or never. The left offensive end blocked down on the defensive tackle, leaving the defensive end on the left side unblocked. As the end moved forward into the offensive back-field, thinking he had been accidently overlooked, Mike Pouncey, the six-foot-five and 312-pound guard, agilely stepped back from the line, turned to the left,

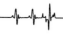

and ran low to ground and parallel to offensive line toward the unsuspecting defensive end (see **Figure 2.4**). Building up a full head of steam, he slammed into the defensive end, hurling him out of the off-tackle hole as his twin brother Maurice led interference through the huge opening in the defensive line that was big enough for a Mack Truck to drive through. Just as the hole opened, the quarterback, Tim Tebow, handed the ball off to running back Percy Harvin, who glided effortlessly and untouched for 52 yards. This beautifully orchestrated play quickly shifted the momentum back to Florida and resulted in a three-point field goal. Florida never looked back, defeating Oklahoma 24-14[1].

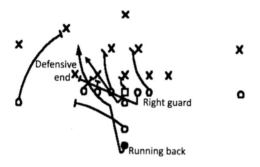

Figure 2.4. University of Florida football traps play. *X*'s indicate the defensive players and *O*'s the offensive players. The square indicates the center. (See text for full explanation.)

What conditions allowed Florida to execute this complex and devastating running play that broke Oklahoma's spirit? First and most importantly, there was no ambiguity regarding each player's assignment. Every player knew where he had to be and what he had to do (see **Figure 2.4**). Second, the timing had to be exact. Any mistake in timing could have resulted in one or more players bumping into each other or the hole closing before the running back reached the line of scrimmage. Everyone had to move quickly and simultaneously. Third, the working relationships between the offensive team members had to be stable. The quarterback had to feel comfortable handing off to the running back, and each lineman had to be familiar with the running speed of the other linemen and the running back.

If a new player had been substituted prior to such a complex play, the probability of an error in timing and coordination would have increased. Having the same teammates work together for the entire season ensures the highest performance. The longer teams are together, the better their performance. The fourth condition that made Florida successful was the players learned each play by doing. To perfect the trap play the team had to practice the specific movements in the play 40 to 50 times before their timing was perfected. Fifth, the players received constant feedback from their coaches. Coaches made suggestions to allow the team to continually improve. This great team made small improvements every day. They never stopped getting better, and by bowl season, they were in peak form.

Key Lessons from the UF Football Team

- There can be no ambiguity regarding individual assignments.

- Everyone needs to understand his/her specific roles.

- Timing of all processes needs to be carefully orchestrated and any wasted time eliminated.

- The working relationships between team members need to be well established and stable.

- Perfect performance requires continual practice.

- Coaching allows the team to continually reflect on their performance and to continually ask the following two questions:
  - What is working well?
  - What can be improved?

Health care providers need to keep in mind these important lessons. Everyone must understand their exact roles within the team. Everyone must respect the importance of timing, and continually work to eliminate all processes and actions that waste time. Once a care team has formed, it is important to establish stability and not constantly rotate members in and

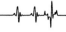

out of the team because continual substitutions increase the likelihood of errors due to unreliable handoffs and poor communication. Teamwork is best learned by working together under the guidance of a coach who provides continual feedback and encourages the team to continually ask, "What is working well, and what can be improved?"

The Three Practices that Create Championship Athletic Teams and the Highest Quality Health Care

What are the basic practices that led to both of these championship athletic teams' successes? Just like high performing industries, these teams successfully followed three key practices: playbooks, knowing who is receiving the ball, and game films.

1. Playbooks

As shown in **Figure 2.4**, the coach designs detailed diagrams that describe exactly where each player should be positioned during the play. Each play represents a compilation of years of trial and errors that have led to the most efficient and effective way of achieving a score. In practice, the players run through each play in slow motion under the guidance of their coaches, and once the coaches are assured that their movements are accurate, the play is run full speed without an opposing defense. Once the coaches are assured that the players are correctly performing the play at full speed, they add defensive opposition.

After the offense has learned a series of plays using the slow motion, full speed without opposition, full speed with opposition cycle, they are ready to scrimmage, and the ideal scrimmage should simulate the intensity of a real game. Early in the season players carry their playbooks everywhere as they memorize their plays. As they look over each play, many of the most successful players visualize their movements and imagine running the play during the upcoming game. Visualization helps to ingrain the proper motor skills and increases the likelihood of a perfect performance.

Curiously, nursing students rarely perform such exercises. They primarily focus on factual content and to a lesser extent on problem solving.

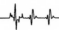

As a consequence, spaghetti motion diagrams of "fully-trained" nursing movements reveal excessive motion on rounds and in the clinic that waste both time and effort. As shown in **Figure 2.5**, the walking paths of a nurse in charge of four patients in rooms 1, 3, 6, and 7 can be plotted over time. As you can see, over two hours this nurse was constantly running between the rooms. On two occasions she was required to leave the immediate area, walking to the right end of the hallway to pick up a supply in the linen closet and to the left to retrieve a bedside commode. Spaghetti diagrams allow documentation of the distance a nurse walks during a specific time period. Medical-surgical nurses walk an average three miles during a ten-hour shift[24]. By providing supplies at the bedside and assigning nurses to care for patients in adjacent rooms, walking distances can be shortened, which would reduce physical effort and increase the time the nurse can spend with each patient. Playbooks that incorporate best practices, simulation exercises, and coaching have the potential to improve efficiency and reduce physical stress.

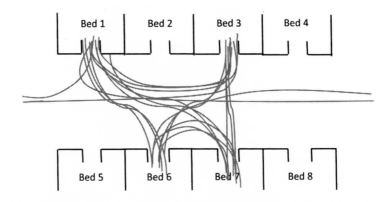

Figure 2.5. Spaghetti diagram. This diagram shows the walking paths of a hospital ward nurse over a two-hour period.

2. Knowing who is passing and who is receiving the ball

In business this is called the customer-supplier relationship. In athletics this is one of the most critical determinants of team success. Error-free passing and catching requires that each team member understand the other's abilities and preferences.

In volleyball, the setter must know how each hitter prefers to have the ball positioned to maximize the force of the hitter's striking motion. The setter is supplying the perfect ball position for the hitter, and when the setter is successful, the probability of a kill is maximized. In order to achieve this goal, the setter and hitter must communicate and iteratively adjust their play until the ideal position is achieved.

Similarly in football, the passer must be familiar with the abilities and preferences of those receiving the ball. As discussed earlier, too many of our passing-catching and handoff relationships in medicine are dysfunctional. By imagining we are passing or handing off to another provider, we will be reminded of the importance of interactive communication and stable relationships. These interactions should not be taken for granted. Just like the setter in volleyball or the quarterback in football, caregivers must practice, practice, practice to continually improve how they communicate and coordinate the care of their patients.

3. Game films

During the heat of battle, events occur quickly, and there is little chance to learn and improve. Recognizing this reality, coaches set aside time after each game to review the team's performance and assess what went well and what could be improved. Usually within twenty-four hours of each game, the coaches and players review the films of the game. Each play is analyzed first by the coaches, and then both the best and worst plays are selected for review with the players.

The coaches point out outstanding techniques that led to the successful plays, allowing all the players to learn from these successes. Individual players are verbally rewarded for their performances. For plays in which errors are observed, the coaches explain to the individual players how they can improve. Often such errors are the consequence of missed assignments, mistiming, or poor fundamental technique. Game films provide feedback for the entire team, and when accompanied by the constructive suggestions for improvement, they allow performance to continually improve.

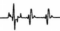

There are several important principles exemplified by game films. First, performance should be assessed within a short period. Otherwise just like fresh fruit, the memories of the performance will fade; feedback will have less meaning and will be less likely to generate significant improvements in performance. Second, the entire team can learn from an open discussion of both the successes and failures of individual team members.

In health care, nursing and physician performances are reviewed only when there is a serious error. Successes in performance are rarely discussed or recognized. Because of their negative focus, morbidity and mortality conferences are often viewed as punitive. Furthermore, these conferences are usually convened weeks to months after the error and/or complication has occurred, greatly reducing the learning opportunities.

Health care providers should consider holding weekly conferences that review not only the failures but also the successes of the care delivery teams. Successful athletes acknowledge that they are error prone and are open to constructive criticism because they recognize that by learning from their error, they can improve their performance and increase the likelihood of victory. In contrast, physicians believe they should be perfect, and any error is considered a shameful embarrassment. Too often they blame others, including nurses. Shame encourages secrecy and causes many caregivers to hide their errors. When errors are hidden, no one can learn from these mistakes, and these errors are likely to be repeated over and over again. Until physicians and nurses develop a game-film approach to their mistakes, there can be no improvement.

All athletes accept and embrace the fact that their play is transparent to the fans. Players love the cheers when they succeed and accept the silence of their fans when a play fails. Referees use a whistle to notify everyone when an error has occurred, and every mistake is acknowledged by a penalty. However, unlike health care providers, players understand that mistakes are part of the game, and they use these errors as opportunities to improve. Everyone in health care needs to embrace a similar transparency and openness. They need to openly acknowledge all mistakes and learn from them.

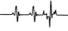

Key Practices of Championship Athletic and Health Care Teams
1. Playbooks
   - All processes and individual players' roles in those processes must be carefully spelled out.
   - Training begins with slow simulation, then full speed simulation, and finally full speed on the wards or in the clinic.

2. Knowing who is passing and who is catching
   - Stable relationships are critical.
   - There must be continual communication between the passer and receiver.
   - Each must understand the strengths and weaknesses of the other.

3. Game films
   - Performance is reviewed within twenty-four hours to avoid memory loss and event spoilage.
   - Successes and failures of individual teammates should be shared openly to allow everyone to learn and improve.
   - Hiding errors prevents learning and ensures the errors will be repeated.

Applying Athletic Principles to Multidisciplinary Rounds

As an attending physician on the inpatient service, I attempted to improve work rounds. Originally I used Toyota and car manufacturing analogies; however, my fellow physicians failed to identify with automobile manufacturing. While watching the University of Florida win the NCAA National Football Championship game on television, I became upset when one of our linemen jumped offsides at a critical point in the game. I yelled out, "Systems error!" It was at that moment that I instantly understood that athletics could serve as superb analogy for the manufacturing principles utilized by Toyota Production System.

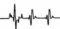

The very next day, I created playbooks that describe the roles of each member of the rounding team using analogies from volleyball, football, and basketball. The playbook designates the attending physician as the head coach, and he or she supervises the team, ensures that all members of the team are effectively following the plays, and continually helps the team members to improve their performance. The nurses are the offensive line, and without their contribution, it would be impossible for the team to succeed. This analogy emphasizes the critical role of the nurses on the team. The team resident is the setter, quarterback, or point guard, serving to distribute the patients to the interns and to call the plays with assistance of the coach. This analogy makes it clear that the coach and the quarterback must continually communicate. The interns are the running backs who carrying the ball; that is, they have direct responsibility for the day-to-day care of each patient. The medical students are redshirt freshman whose primary role is to learn how to play the game. Finally, the case manager and pharmacist are both designated assistant coaches who assist the head coach and team in managing patient disposition and ensuring that medications are properly administered by the nurses.

Just as in a game, the rounding team continually forms a circular huddle where everyone is encouraged to participate in creating each patient's game plan. Just as the offensive coach prepares a series of plays in advance that will be run at the beginning of the game, the attending and team resident together plan out morning work rounds the prior evening, establishing approximate times when each patient will be seen and relaying this schedule to the bedside nurses. Creation of a rounding schedule allows the nurses to plan their morning and allocate time to actively participate on rounds.

Our preliminary pilot program, called *Gatorounds*, has demonstrated a significant improvement in nurses' sense of respect regarding their interactions with physicians, an increased desire on the part of physicians to include nurses in their work rounds deliberations, shortened hospital stays, and a reduced percentage of patients requiring readmission to the hospital. (see http://gatorounds.med.ufl.edu for additional details, accessed 12/20/10).

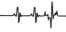

Key Points about Using Athletic Principles for Multidisciplinary Rounds

- Using football, volleyball, and basketball analogies can enable the creation of clear role definitions for each member of the team:
  - Attending physician = coach
  - Team resident = quarterback, point guard, setter
  - Intern = running back, forward, hitter
  - Medical student = redshirt freshman
  - Nurses = the offensive line
  - Case manager and pharmacist = assistant coaches

- Continually huddling—the coach encouraging everyone including the bedside nurse to participate in creating game plans for each patient—is critical.

- Plays are drawn out before rounds; specific times scheduled for bedside rounds allow nurses to participate.

- Consistent implementation of the program improves nurses' sense of respect from physicians, encourages nurse participation, can shorten length of stay, and reduces thirty-day readmissions.

Conclusions about Athletics and Health Care

Athletics provides many of the same guiding principles as the Toyota Production System and Southwest Airlines and allows health care providers to more readily understand these principles. Athletic teams also exemplify the ideals of true teamwork. When our athletic coaches faithfully apply these guiding principles, their teams often achieve national preeminence. Don't patients and health care providers deserve the same high-quality systems as our athletic teams?

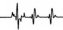

References

1. Jody Hoffer Gittell. 2003. The Southwest Airlines way: Using the power of relationships to achieve high performance. New York: McGraw-Hill.

2. Airsafe.Com. 2011. *Airlines with No Fatal Plane Crashes Since 1970* [Website] 2011 [cited October 6, 2011 2011]. Available from http://www.airsafe.com/events/nofatals.htm.

3. T. Ohno. 1988. *Toyota Production System: Beyond large-scale production.* Portland, OR: Productivity Press.

4. E. S. Fisher, J. P. Bynum, and J. S. Skinner. 2009. Slowing the growth of health care costs--lessons from regional variation. *N Engl J Med* 360 (9):849-852.

5. A. A. Gawande. 2009. The Cost Conundrum. *The New Yorker.*

6. D. M. Berwick. 2010. *Crossing the Quality Chasm: Health Care in the 21st Century.* Cambridge, MA: Institute of Healthcare Improvement.

7. K. D. Calligaro. 2010. Do no harm. *J Vasc Surg* 51 (2):487-493.

8. J.K. Liker, and D. Meier. 2006. *The Toyota Way Field Manual.* New York, NY: McGraw-Hill.

9. J.K. Liker, and M. Hoseus. 2008. *Toyota Culture.* New York, NY: McGraw-Hill.

10. J. G. Nooney, L. Unruh, and M. M. Yore. 2010. Should I stay or should I go? Career change and labor force separation among registered nurses in the U.S. *Soc Sci Med* 70 (12):1874-1881.

11. Richard M. J. Bohmer. 2009. *Designing care : aligning the nature and management of health care.* Boston, Mass.: Harvard Business Press.

12. N. John, G. V. Murthy, P. Vashist, and S. K. Gupta. 2008. Work capacity and surgical output for cataract in the national capital region of Delhi and neighbouring districts of north India. *Indian J Public Health* 52 (4):177-184.

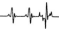
13. Michael E. Porter, and Elizabeth Olmsted Teisberg. 2006. *Redefining health care : creating value-based competition on results*. Boston, Mass.: Harvard Business School Press.

14. S. J. Spear, and H.K. Bowmen. 1999. Decoding the DNA of the Toyota Production System. *Harv Bus Rev* (September-October Issue):1-12.

15. E. G. Van Eaton, K. Mcdonough, W. B. Lober, E. A. Johnson, C. A. Pellegrini, and K. D. Horvath. 2010. Safety of using a computerized rounding and sign-out system to reduce resident duty hours. *Acad Med* 85 (7):1189-1195.

16. K. M. Haig, S. Sutton, and J. Whittington. 2006. SBAR: a shared mental model for improving communication between clinicians. *Joint Commission journal on quality and patient safety / Joint Commission Resources* 32 (3):167-175.

17. D. Pothier, P. Monteiro, M. Mooktiar, and A. Shaw. 2005. Pilot study to show the loss of important data in nursing handover. *British journal of nursing* 14 (20):1090-1093.

18. E. G. Van Eaton, K. D. Horvath, W. B. Lober, and C. A. Pellegrini. 2004. Organizing the transfer of patient care information: the development of a computerized resident sign-out system. *Surgery* 136 (1):5-13.

19. K. H. Gamble. 2010. Wireless Tech Trends 2010. Trend: smartphones. *Healthc Inform* 27 (2):24, 26-27.

20. V. Rich, P.J. Brenan, K. Williams, E. Riley-Wasserman, and L. May. 2008. Clinical leadership on the unit and at the top— a "Swiss Army knife" for sustained performance. Paper read at University of Pennsylvania Health System Consortium, Qualtiy and Safety Fall Forum, at Philadelphia, PA.

21. J.W. Carvin. 2005. *A Piece of the Pie: The Story of Customer Service at Publix*. Kearney, NE: Morris Publishing Co.

22. F. Southwick. 2009. Unpublished personal observations.

23. M. Wise. 2005. Competitiveness. In *She Can Coach!* Champaign, IL: Human Kinetics.

24. A. Hendrich, M. Chow, B.A. Skierczynski, and Z. Lu. 2008. A 36-Hospital Time and Motion Study: How do medical-surgical nurses spend their time? *Permanente J* 12:25-34.

Chapter 2 Exercises

1. As a patient, have you experienced a wasteful process? If so, how would you improve this process? Ask why five times before designing a potential improvement.

2. In your own life, is everything you do of value in achieving your goals?

    a. Remembering the eight forms of waste, list ideas of how you could reduce waste in your life.

    b. Do you adhere to schedules and playbooks? If so, describe them in detail. If not why not?

3. What are your customer-supplier relationships?

    a. Could they be improved?

    b. Are they stable?

4. Do you have a web of close working relationships in your workplace? Explain.

5. Do you experience joy at work? Why or why not?

6. At work, do you share the ball or are you a ball hog?

    a. Are you the point guard, or is there someone else who serves this role?

    b. Are there ways you could distribute the responsibility and work more evenly?

7. Do you apply game films in your life?

    a. How often do you reflect on your daily activities?

    b. How often do you review what went well?

    c. How often to you ask what could be improved?

    d. Do you feel you are open to change?

e.   Do you make errors and mistakes?

f.   Describe several mistakes.

g.   If you are perfect, please explain. We all would like to learn from your best practices.

–3–

MANAGING THE GAME PLAN

What Can the Patient Safety and
Quality Movement Tell Us about Mary's Care?

Guiding Questions

1. What do we mean by quality, and how does quality relate to safety?

2. What is the definition of a system, and how do systems affect quality?

3. What do variability and reliability have to do with safety?

4. What analytic methods can help to differentiate random change from true improvement?

5. Why are human errors so common, and what conditions increase the likelihood of human errors?

6. What are root cause analysis and plan-do-study-act cycles?

7. What is a forcing function?

8. How do you assess a health care system's safety climate?

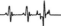

Lost Opportunities

Experts in quality and safety emphasize listening to the patient and the family's concerns. If the system where Mary was cared for had had a strong patient-first culture, the concerns I expressed as a family member and fellow caregiver would have been acted upon much more quickly. A strong quality and safety culture fosters multidisciplinary teams that encourage extensive communication between nurses and physicians, as well as other caregivers. A highly functional multidisciplinary team would have quickly identified the underdosing of Mary's blood thinner. The use of carefully designed treatment protocols for standard treatments is another approach emphasized by safety experts, and as discussed in the previous chapter on TPS, such a protocol could also have prevented the underdosing of Mary's blood thinner. The combination of improved communication and protocols provides multiple fail-safe points to prevent errors. Effective coordination of services is another important safety and quality principle that had the potential to bring together the many subspecialists to create a useful combined set of recommendations that would have encouraged earlier treatment with corticosteroids.

What Do We Mean by Quality?

For the decade after World War II, Japanese-manufactured products were synonymous with low quality. I remember my grandmother buying me a Japanese manufactured toy aircraft carrier. The huge toy was bright and appealing, but within two hours the crank-operated plane elevator had broken because of defective cog alignment. Next, the above-deck superstructure detached from the main ship. Then the toy plane propellers fell off after one or two attempts at spinning them. My initial joy and excitement quickly turned to disappointment. I personally experienced the reality of early post-WWII Japanese products. They malfunctioned or broke far more frequently than products manufactured in other industrialized countries.

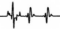

When it comes to defining *quality*, this noun has an amazing number of dimensions, and these dimensions change depending on the product or service you are talking about. In the case of my toy, the quality dimensions that became immediately apparent were performance, reliability, and durability. When it comes to health care, the most important dimension of quality is safety, and because it is deemed the most vital characteristic of quality, *safety* is included as a separate noun. Hospital systems are now appointing chief quality and safety officers, and many systems include improving quality and safety as primary goals.

Another important dimension of quality is aesthetics, and in my case this was the only dimension where the Japanese had achieved a high-quality score. Having this quality characteristic alone can lead to extreme customer dissatisfaction. Imagine yourself being attracted to and buying a product because you found it aesthetically pleasing, and then once you brought it home, you discovered it performed unreliably and quickly fell apart. As a child, I never forgot the bitter disappointment of my toy aircraft carrier, and for years whenever I saw the words *made in Japan* on a toy and my mother asked me if she should buy it, I responded with a deep frown and an emphatic, "No thanks." Similarly, nurses and patients need to understand that just because a hospital has a beautiful lobby does not mean the medical care will be of high quality, and later in this chapter we will discuss the key quality measures that each of us should investigate before trusting our lives to a health care system.

Just like beauty, quality is in the eye of the beholder, the customer, or—in the case of a hospital—the patient. Today product designs are often based on rigorous customer surveys that help define the quality dimensions for each product and service. Health systems are beginning to do the same. Patient satisfaction surveys and suggestions for improvement are now an integral part of all hospitals and clinics that are truly devoted to improving the quality of their care. If the health system that you work in is not asking patients to fill out surveys to assess their needs, likes, and dislikes, you should work with your administration to improve their patient focus.

> **Key Points about Quality and Safety**
> - Quality has many dimensions, including reliability, performance, durability, efficiency, and safety.
>
> - Aesthetics should not be ignored; however, aesthetics in the absence of performance and reliability can result in great frustration.

What Role Do Systems Play in Quality?

The Japanese quickly realized that they would never achieve economic prosperity if they could not improve the quality of their exports. To this end, they embraced the teachings of the American W. Edwards Deming, who combined the theories of systems, the understanding of variation, the building of knowledge, and an appreciation for human behavior to show how companies could continually improve their products and services.

Deming knew that improving systems operation was the key to improving the manufacturing quality. Similarly, systems improvements are critical for improving the quality of patient care. I know when I first heard the word *care system*, I cringed and thought to myself, *What's this system junk? This has nothing to do with my patients.* I imagined complex computations and MIT engineers. I didn't understand because I was unaware how well-designed systems could dramatically improve health care delivery (i.e., quality). Only after learning of the remarkable accomplishments of Toyota Production Systems did I realize that systems were the key to preventing other patients from suffering Mary's fate[1].

What is a system? A system can be defined as an interdependent group of items, people, or processes working together toward a common purpose[2].By this definition, an athletic team and a health team are both systems. However, it gets more complicated than that. A group of health care teams working within a hospital or clinic is also a system, as is a group of hospitals and clinics working together for a common purpose. Our state governments and our federal government are systems. In fact, we encounter systems all day, every day. When we turn on a light, we are benefiting from an electrical system. When we eat at a restaurant, we are benefiting from a food delivery system. I could go on and on.

As I first thought about this definition, I began to realize that the ultimate success of any organization, including car manufacturing and health care, depends on the integration of all the individual parts. Because these parts are interdependent—that is, they are attached physically or functionally to one another—when you adjust one part, you will usually need to simultaneously adjust other parts. In other words, when it comes to systems, changes usually have to occur simultaneously in multiple areas in order to effectively improve the function of the entire system.

In integrated systems, it also true that if one part malfunctions, this event will typically lead to the dysfunction of other parts within the system. As a very simple example, let's examine an electric toy train set. (In case you hadn't noticed, I loved toys as a child.) Let's make it one of those big Lionel train sets with the crossing gates, a sleek, black, smoking engine, ornate passenger cars, and last but not least, a bright red caboose. What happens if the wheels on the caboose freeze up? As the engine pulls the train, the caboose wheels squeak, and the caboose begins to shake from side to side. The engine begins to overheat because of the increased workload. You happen to be talking to a friend on the phone, and you fail to notice these events. The side-to-side shaking of the caboose increases and spreads to the adjacent passenger cars, the train derails, breaking the delicate crossing gate, and you discover that the electrical engine has burned out. This simple example illustrates how the malfunctioning of one part can eventually lead to systems failure, and unfortunately in health care, there are malfunctioning parts and systems failures everywhere.

What would have happened if you had been carefully monitoring the train as it sped along its tracks and you had immediately noticed the caboose's squeaking wheels and shut down the train? You would have discovered that the wheel axles had become rusty in the damp basement where your parents insisted you store your train set. You then could have lubricated the axles until they spun smoothly. This intervention would have restored normal function and prevented the damage to your train set. You would have saved an expensive engine repair bill, as well as the purchase price of a new crossing gate. Are you beginning to understand the concepts of system malfunction, diagnosis, and correction? The key ingredients are quite simple: a full understanding of your system and well-honed common sense.

Systems are not usually as simple as a toy train, and they do not usually consist of simple linear, sequential connections. Health care and manufacturing systems can be very complex and may require experts in systems analysis to detect and correct the systems defects in order to prevent systems failure. However, many of the smaller and simpler systems of medicine, sometimes called microsystems, can be analyzed and corrected using everyday common sense, just like our Lionel train set.

To get an idea of what I am talking about in health care, let's take look at an example of a poorly functioning microsystem in Mary's case. The neurologist who first saw Mary had created a system for caring for his patients. He had an office that included a small waiting room, an examining room with a table, and procedure room containing a machine that measured nerve conduction velocity. To manage the clinic, he employed an appointment and reception secretary, a technician who performed the nerve conduction studies, and a part-time nurse who assisted him on his clinic days. He had no other physician partners in his clinic. The secretary and technician both depended on him to care for the patients, to dictate when a patient would return, and to decide who would receive an electrical conduction study. The overall goal of this interdependent group was to diagnose and treat peripheral nerve injuries.

Unfortunately for Mary, his simple clinic system was flawed because it had no built-in contingency plans for patient care when the sole caregiver left town. On the days when he was away, whenever a patient called requesting immediate neurological care as I did for Mary, his secretary simply told the patient he was out of town. Thus the system simply shut down when he was away.

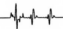

What could have happened if his clinic system had been functioning properly? This system defect could have been readily corrected by recruiting a second neurologist and establishing the systems rule that both physicians should never be out of town and/or unavailable at the same time. I could have called the clinic, and Mary would have been seen by a second neurologist, and in all likelihood he would have noticed that her nerve pain was then associated with unusual skin lesions, which suggested an immune reaction. He then would have drawn blood tests and found her very high eosinophil count. The findings of a local peripheral nerve injury (called *mononeuritis* by neurologists), eosinophilia (abnormally high numbers of eosinophils, which is seen primarily in allergic reactions), and blood-filled skin lesions (suggesting that Mary's immune system was attacking blood vessels in the skin) would have encouraged him to begin Mary on an oral corticosteroid.

Treatment with this strong anti-inflammatory agent would have prevented further progression of her severe penicillin allergic reaction and prevented her hospitalization. And just as a failure to correct the squeaky caboose wheels eventually leads to an expensive systems failure, in Mary's case the neurologist's defective clinic system made possible multiple additional errors: a near total systems failure of care and Mary's near death. The resulting complications cost far more than a model train repair.

In the business world, the most successful companies produce the highest quality products and services because they have created efficient, error-free production systems. These companies prosper because they are able to attract customers, while those companies whose products are of lower quality go out of business. When it comes to health care systems, the same rules do not apply; however, the rules are beginning to change. If health care consumers could be provided with accurate measures of quality and cost, business experts maintain that health care could also become a truly consumer-driven market, and this condition would reward ever-improving, high-quality health care systems[3].

Most importantly, in addition to providing a competitive financial advantage and attracting more patients, high-functioning systems allow caregivers to

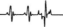

provide better patient care. In modern medicine, the systems of care and the caregiver are interdependent, and patients as well as society regard our systems of care and the caregiver as one. We are a central part of the system. All caregivers must devote time and energy to improving their local systems of care in addition to improving their personal skills.

Key Points about Systems

- A system is an interdependent group of items, people, or processes working together toward a common purpose.

- The malfunctioning of one part of a system will lead to the malfunction of other system parts, which will eventually cause overall system failure.

- Identifying a system malfunction quickly prevents costly system failures.

- Medicine consists of many microsystems amenable to improvement by those working within the system.

- Microsystems improvements usually require only two ingredients: an intimate knowledge of the system and common sense.

- As health care providers, we need to improve our systems in addition to improving our personal skills.

- Today, the system and caregiver are one. We are the central part of the system.

Understanding Variability and Reliability

Quality improvement requires meaningful feedback. Each time we intervene to repair a system, to improve the quality of its output we need to ask the question, "Did my intervention make a difference?" To understand how challenging this question is, we need to return to the lessons of W. Edwards Deming and his teacher, Walter E. Shewhart.

In a recent class, I had the pleasure of partaking in Deming's famous red bead experiment. Dr. Donald Berwick, the former head of IHI and current chief administrator of the center for Medicare Medicaid Services (CMS), came to our classroom with a drum filled with 3200 white beads and 800 red beads—four white beads to every one red bead (see **Figure 3.1**). He asked us to imagine we were the White Bead Manufacturing Company. He selected four students to be his factory workers. Next he trained them how to properly select beads. First he mixed the beads in the drum three times, and then he immersed a plastic spatula with fifty bead pockets into the drum. He then pulled the spatula out of the drum at an approximately 45° angle to ensure all the beads stayed in their holding pockets. Given the mixture of beads, the odds of picking red bead for each well was one in five; therefore, the average number of red beads selected by chance should be ten out of fifty.

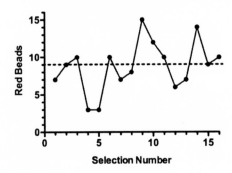

Red Bead Experiment

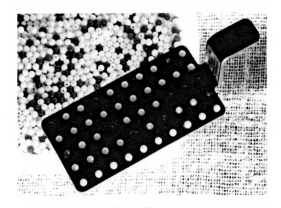

Figure 3.1. Red bead experiment (see text for details)

Dr. Berwick next appointed a supervisor and told the supervisor that the White Bead Manufacturing Company was trying to reduce the number of red beads in their selection process and that the selection of a red bead was considered an error. The goal for each worker should be to capture six or less red beads per selection try. Workers who achieved this goal would receive a bonus. Any worker selecting more than ten red beads would be placed on probation. (Based on our understanding of odds ratio for picking a red bead, these goals were unfair.) The supervisor was assigned to count the number of red beads in each selection try.

Despite carefully following Dr. Berwick's directions and performing the selection procedure in a consistent and careful manner, only three of the workers' sixteen tries yielded red ball counts of less than six, and two students were placed on probation for repeatedly selecting ten or more red beads. Dr. Berwick then asked the participants how it felt to work in this bead factory. Student workers volunteered that they were frustrated and defensive about their performance and felt no sense of control. As time went on, they became increasingly resentful of the company's unrealistic and impossible expectations and also became fearful about losing their jobs.

The student designated as supervisor felt he had no control over his workers or the bead selection process. Because he was directly watching them while they selected the beads, he assumed the workers were personally to blame for the "poor" performance. As the supervisor, he focused on the people, the bonuses, and the probation. He was disappointed in everyone's poor performance and wanted to be supportive to his workers, but he was forced to follow the rules of the company. He felt caught in the middle.

When everyone stepped backed and examined the experiment, they began laughing. They realized that the variations in red bead numbers were strictly the consequence of random chance and that the workers could not reduce the red bead count by simply following the selection procedure dictated by the company. When the students brainstormed together, they quickly realized that the only way to reduce these random "errors" was to remove all the red beads from the drum before they began selecting beads.

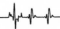

In other words, they had to make a fundamental change in the system to improve the reliability for selecting white beads.

Similarly, many of the systems problems and errors caregivers and patients encounter are the consequence of stable but unacceptably variable processes. Just as the students realized they should not blame each other and instead redesign the process, we need to stop attributing medical errors to people and redesign our frontline care systems to eliminate the errors resulting from random variation. We all need to remove the red beads. *Errors are not caused by bad people, but rather they are caused by bad systems.*

At first, students attributed the selection of red balls to individual behavior, but in reality these differences could be explained by chance. However, not all errors can be explained by chance. In fact, many errors are the result of new defects within a system caused by changes in human behavior or defective equipment, as exemplified by the Lionel train example described earlier. Unfortunately, when it comes to breakdowns in the function of medical systems, they are not as easy to detect as a squeaking wheel. Despite this limitation, just as observed in our train example, it is critical to quickly identify and correct such defects to prevent patient injuries. But how do we differentiate between chance events and events caused by a new defect in the system? And when we redesign a system, how do we know our change has improved the system?

Deming and Shewhart dedicated their careers to creating statistical methods for differentiating common cause (random cause) variation from special cause (caused by a modifiable cause) variation. Common cause variation remains constant or stable over time and is predictable. However, when a special cause is combined with common cause variation, the variation is no longer random and takes on a new pattern. Once the special cause is identified and removed, variation will again become random.

Deming and Shewhart used analytical methods that are very different from the methods usually employed in scientific papers. In classical statistics, all the data of individual experiments are combined or pooled into a single average and the deviation calculated. From the standpoint of quality improvement, this is the equivalent of driving a car forward while looking through the rearview

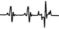

mirror. To provide real-time data that allows timely adjustments, Deming and Shewhart recommended that all quality data be graphically depicted as single points over time, and they rightfully claimed that this method uncovers the "knowledge that lives within the data"[2]. To this end they created two types of time-series plots.

The first and simplest plot is called a run chart. Each quality measure score is plotted as a specific time point, and after fifteen to twenty time points have been accumulated, the data can be analyzed to determine if the variation in score over time is a result of common cause alone or demonstrates special cause variation. First the median or midpoint value for the data is calculated, and a horizontal line is drawn across the graph to represent the median (dashed line in **Figure 3.1**).

Next the number of points above or below the median is counted. Points on the median line should not be counted. A run is one or more points above or below the median. If the run has five points in a row on one side of the median, this is considered a *trend*, while six points in a row indicates a *shift in process*. **Figure 3.1** is a run plot of the red bead experiment described earlier. Note that no trends or runs are observed, and there are equal numbers of points above the median and below the median. This run chart confirms that the differences between the four workers were simply caused by common cause variation (i.e., chance).

How can a run chart be used to analyze a medical system? Work rounds on the inpatient medical service can be highly variable. One very useful way to determine the effectiveness of hospital care is to track the percentage of hospitalized patients who require readmission within thirty days. Readmission is considered a systems failure because rehospitalization indicates that the patient's health problems were not effectively treated. As shown in **Figure 3.2A**, in the absence of any change in the rounding system (control rounding group) the thirty-day readmission rate was predictably variable, indicating common cause variation (equal numbers of points above and below the median). The median readmission rate was 10.8 percent, and I felt that a rounding systems failure rate of worse than one out of ten patients was unacceptable.

As described at the end of the Chapter 2 and in the next chapter (**Case 4.6**), I encouraged the formation of an effective multidisciplinary team that included both bedside nurses and the nurse case manager to improve the coordination of care, and as shown in **Figure 3.2B**, I significantly altered the run chart. Rather than having equal numbers of points above and below the median, as seen in the control group (**Figure 3.2A**), the experimental group shifted eleven of thirteen points below the median and also achieved a run of six points below the median. This run chart demonstrates special cause variation and strongly suggests the intervention significantly reduced the percentage of thirty-day readmissions to the hospital.

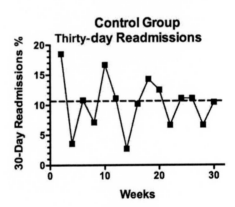

Figure 3.2A. Run chart of the control rounding team

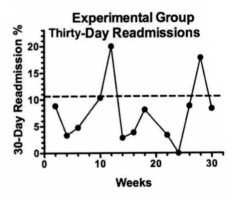

Figure 3.2B. Run chart of the experimental multidisciplinary rounding team (*Gatorounds*)

In addition to run charts, outcome measures can be plotted using a control, or Shewhart plot. In place of simply using the median as the guidepost, this method uses mean and standard deviation calculations to create upper and lower limits for variation. When data exceeds these limitations, it suggests special cause variation. Standard deviation is a method for creating a numerical score that reflects the variability of data. When the swings in values are wide, the standard deviation will be higher; if the data are closely bunched around the median, the standard deviation will be low, and the median value is likely to accurately reflect the true value. The data from the red bead experiment can be replotted as a control chart format (**Figure 3.3**) and shows that the values remain within the two standard deviation limits, indicating variance is a result of common cause.

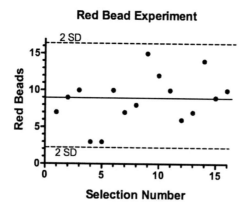

Figure 3.3. Shewhart Plot or Control Chart of the Red Bead Experiment

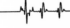

> **Key Points about Variation**
> - All processes are variable, called common cause variation.
>   - This is demonstrated by Deming's red bead experiment.
>   - Often those working on the front lines are personally blamed for common cause variation.
>
> - To assess if there is a new problem within the system or to determine if an intervention resulted in an improvement, we must differentiate *common cause* from *special cause* variation.
>
> - Shewhart and Deming recommend plotting all measurement data over time to uncover the "knowledge that lives within the data."
>   - Run plot—fifteen to twenty points plotted over time
>   - Calculate the median.
>   - Examine all points above and below the median:
>   - Five in a row on one side of the median equals a trend.
>   - Six or more in a row equals a shift in process (special cause variation).
>   - Control chart—fifteen to twenty points plotted over time
>   - Calculate the mean.
>   - Calculate the standard deviation.
>   - Beyond two standard deviations suggests special cause variation.

Errors (Red Beads) in Medicine— Why are There so Many?

Errors are part of all of our lives. For example, when I overwork and become fatigued, I often misplace my car keys and must devote time to trying to track them down. This fatigue-associated unintended act prevents me from achieving my intended outcome: to drive my car to work[4]. When I make this error of commission (that is, when I do the wrong thing by placing my keys in an obscure location), this error will delay my arrival at work and backlog my appointment schedule, inconveniencing everyone I was supposed to meet with that day. Imagine if I am scheduled to work in the clinic that morning. All my patients would be impacted by my error. Without proper contingency plans in the clinic system, my error will disrupt the nurses' routines, as well as the appointment clerk's morning. And worst of all, it will inconvenience my patients. My error will also result in an overcrowded waiting room. The ripple effect goes on and on.

Let's consider a worse scenario. Imagine I have an argument with my wife the night before my clinic. By the way, this virtually never happens because my wife Kathie is one of the most patient and understanding people in the entire world. But to illustrate the problem of human errors, imagine as a consequence of my argument, I become so distracted and upset that I forget I was scheduled to work in the clinic the next morning. I decide to stay home and take a mental health day off from work. This is an error of omission. I fail to perform an important task. Unbeknownst to me, the battery in my pager has died, and I decide not to answer the phone because for the past several days we have been plagued by political campaign phone calls.

The clinic supervisor quickly notices I have not arrived at the clinic. He is unable to contact me and frantically calls my office secretary. He knows that several of my patients have traveled for more than two hours to see me. He also knows that one of my patients is very ill and may require hospital admission. In anticipation of unexpected absences, our office has a back-up system. Physicians are paired and share a cohort of patients. In my case, my colleague and friend Gary is my partner, and he knows all of my patients. He has allotted flexible time this morning to complete paper work in his office. When our secretary calls, he rushes down to the clinic and quickly begins seeing my patients. Our back-up clinic coverage system compensates for my error, and our patients and the clinic staff are largely spared any inconvenience. Of course, Gary is quite annoyed, and the next day I profusely apologize and agree to cover one of his clinics in return.

Upon reflecting on these events and exploring the root causes of my error (failing to attend clinic), I realize that a series of improbable events aligned to cause me to miss clinic. I never argue with my wife; I never need to take a mental health day; I always replace my pager battery when it warns me that the battery is aging; and I usually answer my home phone. But on this one unfortunate day, these never events all happen, and I miss clinic. This has been termed the "Swiss cheese model" for errors. That is, a series of errors or holes all lined up perfectly so that the chain of possible corrections or remedies failed to interrupt the error, causing a major injury or death (see **Figure 3.4**)[5].

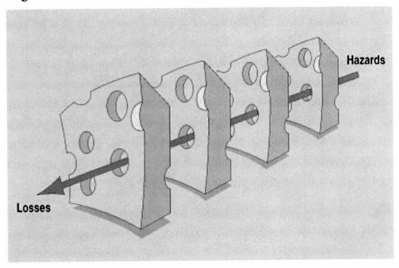

Figure 3.4 The Swiss cheese model of how defenses, barriers, and safeguards may be penetrated by an accident trajectory[5]

When there are poor back-up systems, our patients are in danger. If our clinic back-up system had not been in place and my patients were told to come back another day, imagine the potential fallout. The very sick patient may have returned home, become increasing ill, and required ambulance transport to an emergency room. This patient could have died. The other patients would have become very angry, having driven four hours without receiving the care they expected and needed. As this simple hypothetical example illustrates that hospitals and clinics must design systems to account for human error.

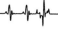

Factors that Increase the Likelihood of Human Errors

The two examples described above illustrate how fatigue and emotional stress can promote errors. We live in a fast-paced world, and too often sleep gets in the way of all the important tasks we need to complete. The Puritan work ethic has made this a particularly acute problem for Americans, and it is estimated that 70 percent of us do not get enough sleep during the week[6]. We now know that adequate sleep is critical for health, and those who get insufficient sleep are more likely to die at a younger age. Sleep deprivation doesn't just affect your health, but it also increases the risk not only of losing your keys but also of having a car accident. Sleep deprivation slows reaction times, and remaining awake for seventeen to nineteen hours slows responses to the same extent as drinking two glasses of beer. Further sleep deprivation results in reaction times comparable to someone with a 0.1 percent blood alcohol level[7, 8], which is over the limit when it comes to drunk driving but not always over the limit for medical providers.

Surveys of night shift nurses have revealed they are twice as likely to make errors and are at greater risk of nodding off at work and while driving. Nurses can employ specific strategies for reducing fatigue and improving performance including: encouraging more than eight hours of sleep before work, implementing strategic twenty-minute naps at work, staffing appropriately to allow complete work and meal breaks, increasing ambient light, avoiding sleep cycle interruptions by frequent changes from day to night shifts, and limiting consecutive as well as total work hours[9, 10]. My wife Kathie now insists that I sleep eight hours per night so that she doesn't have to hear me ask, "Honey, where are my keys?"

Stress resulting from conflicts at home or at work and excessive job demands can combine with sleep deprivation to impair work performance[11]. Human factors research has shown that stressful conditions can increase the chances of an error from 0.1 percent to 30 percent[6]. Health care leaders should be encouraged to create supportive collegial environments not only to improve job satisfaction but also to reduce human errors.

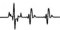

Multitasking is another factor that can exacerbate human error, and as discussed earlier, this was a major factor contributing to the poor performance of the senior physician who first cared for Mary in the hospital. As discussed in Chapter 5, each caregiver must prioritize his or her tasks and complete one task at a time rather than jumping from task to task, trying to advance all tasks simultaneously. Juggling multiple projects inevitably makes one vulnerable to dropping one or more of the balls.

Case 3.1. The medical team gathered for work rounds in the hallway just outside the room of their team's first patient. As the nurse began to present her patient's overnight medical problems, the intravenous infusion pump alarm went off. The nurse paused in her presentation, ran over to the IV pump, discovered the infusion bag was empty, called a fellow nurse to replace the solution bag, and then restarted her presentation. About two sentences into the presentation, her cell phone rang. She again paused and answered the phone. The ward clerk was calling because one of her other patients was requesting a pain medication. After two minutes, the nurse restarted her presentation. By this time, the other members of the team were frustrated and impatient. Ten minutes had passed, and they had barely begun to discuss the first patient.

As described in **Case 3.1**, interruptions occur frequently in health care and can result in incalculable harm. The loss of focus greatly increases the probability of a mistake, and systems that minimize interruption need to be designed. For example, a rule could be established that nurses and physicians will only be contacted for true emergencies during work rounds. All other calls could be held until the completion of rounds. Noise is another major distraction. As interns and nurses present vital information about their patients on rounds, noisy carts are often being wheeled down the hallways, various instrument alarms are sounding, and people too often are talking loudly. Recently my team's work rounds were interrupted by a huge rumbling garbage cart, as well as a noisy floor-waxing machine. A quiet period should be declared on every floor to allow rounds to be conducted in a peaceful supportive environment that encourages caregivers to effectively focus on managing their patients.

Key Points about Human Errors
- We all make errors all the time.

- There are two types of errors:
  - Error of commission—we do the wrong thing.
  - Error of omission—we forget to do something we should have done.

- Errors increase in likelihood with any or all of the following factors:
  - Fatigue—lack of sleep significantly reduces performance (greater than twenty-four hours of sleep deprivation is the equivalent of a blood alcohol level of 0.1 percent)
  - Stress—stress causes reduced mental focus.
  - Multitasking—to minimize errors, one should set priorities and perform one task at a time.
  - Distractions—loud noises and conversations lead to distractions.
  - Interruptions—interruptions are a too common occurrence in medicine.

- Repeated practice and simulation can reduce but never eliminate human errors.
  - Encourage teammates. Don't blame.
  - Call time-outs to develop strategies to prevent errors.

Practice and Simulation Can Reduce but Never Completely Eliminate Errors

As described in Chapter 2, athletes continually practice their plays to reduce errors. Health care providers also need to consciously practice. Simulators and classroom exercises are important venues for practicing key procedures and

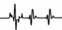

processes. However, in the heat of competition each player makes errors. The most effective players acknowledge their errors and the errors of their fellow teammates. However, rather than blaming others, championship athletes offer encouragement and suggestions to their teammates. They understand that errors are to be expected and recognize that the team that makes the fewest errors wins the game. Whenever a team has a string of errors, the effective athletic coach calls a time-out to discuss the source of the team's mistakes and suggests new strategies to improve performance. Similarly, to reduce errors, caregivers need to take time-outs and huddle to discuss their strategies for improving their performance. Each time an error occurs, just like championship athletic teams, the health care team members need to acknowledge their errors, avoid blame, and encourage everyone to contribute to the team's continual performance improvement.

The Mathematics of Reliability

Mathematicians have also explored the probability of human errors, and there is an entire school of systems design based on the mathematics of errors, called Six Sigma[12]. I know many readers have a phobia when it comes to this subject, but bear with me and you will quickly understand the power of numbers when it comes to human errors. In fact, these concepts relate not only to health care but also to everyday life. Let's assume that particular process can be performed perfectly 99.9 percent of the time. That sounds incredible, doesn't it? That means one out of thousand times, that particular process fails. Quality experts use the term reliability[12]:

$$\text{Reliability} = \frac{\text{Number of actions that achieved the intended result}}{\text{Total number of actions}}$$

Now let's examine the consequences of 99.9 percent reliability when it comes to managing the medications for a patient in the hospital. The average inpatient receives ten medications, and on average these medications are given three times per day. That means individual medications are being administered thirty times per day. Imagine you had to be hospitalized for six days. You would receive medications 180 times during your hospitalization. If the error rate for medication administration is 1/1000, you have approximately a one in five (200/1000 = 1/5) chance of receiving the wrong medication or the wrong dose of a medication. If you were betting in a horse race, those would be considered pretty good odds of winning. But in the case of a hospitalization, you would lose.

The hospital where I work has more than eight hundred beds, and if we extrapolate this mathematical analysis to our entire hospital patient population, this means there will be one hundred and sixty medication errors over an average six-day period. Studies of medication errors reveal that approximately 20 percent of these medication errors will be serious, and about 4 percent of these errors will result in significant harm[13]. Therefore in any six-day period, assuming administration procedures were 99.9 percent accurate, six patients (or one patient per day) would be seriously harmed by a medication administration error. We also know that one out of a hundred serious medication reactions leads to death[13]. Therefore, every one hundred days, one patient would die in our hospital due to a medication error.

Industries such as Toyota and Southwest Airlines realized long ago that 99.9 percent accuracy was unacceptable for their processes, and Six Sigma gets its name from its goal to achieve an error rate of 3.4 per million (3.4 x 10^6, or 99.99966% reliability)[12]. If that is the goal for the manufacturing of automobiles, running nuclear reactors, and piloting airplanes, shouldn't that be the goal for our health care system?

Unfortunately the accuracy of medication ordering and delivery is nowhere close to this 99.9 percent rate in most hospitals. In hospitals where orders are hand written, on average, the error rate is estimated to be 8 percent, rather than 0.1 percent, or 80 times worse[13]. This estimate suggests that in an average eight-hundred-bed hospital that does not employ a computerized ordering system, there will be nearly one death per day due to preventable medication errors! Because nurses are responsible for distributing the majority of medications to patients, those working in systems that continue to rely on handwritten orders and prescriptions are at great risk of inadvertently harming their patients.

To make matters even more worrisome, 99.9 percent is the accuracy of a single step: the nurse handing the medication to the patient. Of course there are multiple steps required before this step. In fact, in most hospitals there are on average more than thirty steps between the ordering of a medication and its distribution. Therefore when you multiply 0.999 by 0.999, thirty times the expected percentage of medications that would be accurately distributed is reduced to 97 percent, which equates to a 3 percent error rate.

The problem of too many steps also applies when we book airline flights. Whenever possible, passengers should try to book a direct flight because if the on-time percentage for the flight is 80 percent, there is an eight-out-of-ten chance of arriving on time. With a direct flight, even if the plane is a little late, there are no connections to miss and unless the flight is canceled, passengers are sure to arrive at their destination. What happens when the flight requires a connection to a second plane with an 80 percent on time record? Now the chances of arriving on time drop to 64 percent (0.8 x 0.8).

I hope this example makes it clear that when it comes to efficiency and reducing errors, the fewer steps the better. As a caregiver, always ask yourself, "What unnecessary steps can I eliminate?" Just as in all of life, those of us working in health care should try to keep it simple. Because of the low reliability of our processes, on average one in ten patients suffers one adverse event during their hospital stay[6]. Rather than being six sigma, our average reliability is one sigma! As experts in systems engineering have repeatedly observed, we have plenty of room for improvement.

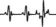

> **Key Points about the Mathematics of Errors**
>
> - Reliability $= \dfrac{\text{Number of actions that achieved the intended result}}{\text{Total number of actions}}$
>
> - Many processes in medicine are unreliable:
>   - Medication errors can be as high as 8 percent.
>   - Adverse events occur in one out of ten inpatients.
>   - When it comes to reliability for medications, even 99.9 percent is unacceptable; we need to aim for six sigma (3.4 error per million).
>
> - Simplification by reducing process steps is a powerful approach to improving reliability.

Tools for Reducing Errors and Improving Reliability

Case 3.2A. Mr. J., a sixty-year-old mechanic, is admitted to the intensive care unit with severe pneumonia. Intravenous antibiotics are begun; however, despite this treatment his blood pressure begins to fall. The ICU physician orders treatment with intravenous norepinephrine, an agent that constricts blood vessels and increases blood pressure. The very busy ICU nurse receives the solution bag containing norepinephrine, as well as a second bag containing the next dose of cefepime, one of the antibiotics used to treat Mr. J's pneumonia. While carrying the medication bags to his bedside, the nurse is paged. She sets both bags down on the bedside table and answers her page. Upon returning, she inadvertently places the norepinephrine bag on the IV pole intended for the antibiotic infusion and places the antibiotic bag on the poll intended for the norepinephrine infusion. As a consequence of this switch, norepinephrine is infused at the much faster rate designated for the antibiotic. The patient's blood pressure rises acutely, and his heart begins beating irregularly, leading to a cardiac arrest and death. The error is not discovered until Mr. J. has died.

Case 3.2A illustrates the worst possible outcome of a human error. Mary also received norepinephrine to raise her blood pressure. Fortunately for us, the ICU physician and nurses remained at her bedside and repeatedly checked the infusion rate of each of her medications, preventing a similar fatal error.

In one popular patient safety book, the word *error* is used 641 times[14], and all safety experts have been intensely focusing on eliminating all errors. Like Mary's case, Mr. J. exemplifies in personal terms the urgency of improving the reliability of care at the bedside. As this case starkly illustrates, a single error can mean the difference between life and death.

Root Cause Analysis (RCA)

One of the most useful tools for investigating sentinel events, that is an event that warns a health care system that there is a serious systems defect, is called root cause analysis or RCA. **Case 3.2A** would be considered a *sentinel event* and would precipitate an intense root cause analysis in virtually all hospitals. This same exercise occurs after a plane crash. Investigators immediately descend on the crash site and gather all the evidence. Evidence related to a serious medical error needs to be gathered immediately before the details fade from the participants' memories. As noted earlier, memories associated with a sentinel event quickly fade.

A root cause analysis requires a careful and specific series of steps:

1. *Recruit an RCA team*—In this case, a critical care physician, an intensive care nurse, a pharmacist, and an expert in facilitating RCAs should be included. The joint commission (the organization that monitors hospital quality) also recommends that a family member be included. Participation of the family not only has the potential to help their healing process, but it also reduces the likelihood of punitive legal action. When the hospital demonstrates a strong will to learn and make corrective changes, family members are assured their loved ones did not die in vain. The family's inclusion also fosters trust and ensures full transparency.

2. *Define the specific goal of the team*—In **Case 3.2A**, the goal would be preventing intravenous medication administration errors.

3. *Intensely study the problem and determine exactly what happened*—To accomplish this, the RCA team needs to
    a. identify all contributing factors and
    b. collect all data related to the problem.

4. *Design and implement a temporary fix*—In the **Case 3.2A** all nurses would be required to administer only one intravenous medication at a time.

5. *Determine the root causes*—This can be a very labor intensive process that requires digging deep and asking why five times.

6. *Initiate a series of plan-do-study-act cycles (PDSA cycles) to create a more permanent solution*—Need to involve frontline caregivers with first hand knowledge of all the procedures.

Let's review the details of **Case 3.2A** to better understand what went wrong. The conditions for making a human error were all in place. The nurse was fatigued and stressed primarily as a consequence of difficulties in her home life. She had a daughter who was failing high school, and they had had an argument, causing her to sleep fitfully the night before the event. Second, she was managing a second ICU patient who also required considerable attention. This assignment necessitated that she run back and forth between the two rooms. To make matters worse, she was paged by one of the physicians about her other patient in the middle of her most important task: hanging the norepinephrine. At the time of the page, she had performed a medication check to ensure that the doses of the two drugs were correct. In order to respond to the page, she set down the two bags, answered the page, and then neglected to recheck the medications before hanging them on the wrong poles. The two bags and the two solutions looked identical, with the exception of the small print describing the content of each bag. There were no identifying labels on the intravenous tubing that could have warned her that she was inserting the norepinephrine line into the antibiotic administration pump.

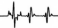

As previously described, the holes in the Swiss cheese slices had aligned (**Figure 3.4**): the nurse was fatigued and stressed, she was required to multitask, two important medications needed to be administered simultaneously and the two medication bags were identical in size and color, and she was interrupted in the middle of administering the medications. She was a victim of poorly designed systems that failed to minimize human error. The systems of care in the ICU failed to prevent a series of small overlapping events from culminating in a fatal error.

Plan-Do-Study-Act (PDSA) Cycles

As described in Chapter 2, many industries employ plan-do-study-act cycles to improve their systems (**Figure 3.5**). When utilizing this very powerful and effective tool for improving reliability, the first question that needs to be asked is, "What are we trying to accomplish?" A very specific goal needs to be created for every PDSA cycle because in the absence of a specific measurable goal, the second important question cannot be answered: "How will we know the change is an improvement?"

For **Case 3.2A**, the goal of the PDSA cycle is to eliminate intravenous medication errors in the intensive care unit. To assess whether or not this goal is achieved, a pharmacist will be assigned to review the administration of all intravenous medications each day. The number of medication errors per one hundred intravenous medications administered (number of errors/one hundred administrations) will be plotted daily using a run chart. The reliability of IV administration can also be plotted daily by dividing the number of errors by the total number of IV medications administered (number of errors ÷ total number of IV administrations).

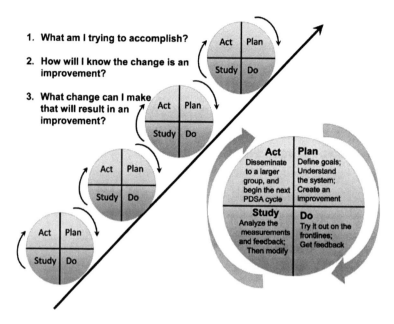

1. **What am I trying to accomplish?**

2. **How will I know the change is an improvement?**

3. **What change can I make that will result in an improvement?**

Act
Disseminate to a larger group, and begin the next PDSA cycle

Plan
Define goals; Understand the system; Create an improvement

Study
Analyze the measurements and feedback; Then modify

Do
Try it out on the frontlines; Get feedback

Figure 3.5. Plan-do-study-act (PDSA) cycles for improvement. See text for details.

Plan

Once the first two questions are answered, the third question should be, "What change can I make that will result in improvement?" To answer this all-important question, there must be careful planning, and this is the first step in the PDSA cycle. Before plans can be created, the team needs to achieve a full understanding of the underlying causes or drivers of the error.

One of the most effective methods for achieving this goal is to ask why five times. Applying the five whys to **Case 3.2A**, the team should ask:

1. Why did the nurse switch the two intravenous medications? Answer: because the two bags looked alike and the labels had small black print.

2. Why? Answer: because an automatic printer prints out all labels.

3. Why? Answer: because this approach saves time and is simple.

4. Why? Answer: because simplicity and efficiency are emphasized by the

director of the pharmacy.

5. Why? Answer: because the pharmacy director prides himself in eliminating all wasteful steps in medication management.

The five whys explain why the pharmacy uses a small-print uniform labeling system, and this new understanding will allow the improvement team to suggest an effective intervention. The good news is that the director of the pharmacy is systems oriented, and his goals to simplify and reduce waste were well meaning. However, this sentinel event warns him that he has oversimplified medication labeling and will need to design a more sophisticated classification and labeling system to alert nurses and physicians when they are administering potentially dangerous drugs.

Using this approach to fully understand what went wrong and why, multiple drivers can be identified and then categorized as primary or secondary. In **Case 3.2A**, the primary drivers and secondary drivers include the following factors (see **Figure 3.6**):

1. Fatigue
   a. Conflict with her daughter
   b. Inability to control stress
   c. Difficulty sleeping
   d. Poor family support by her husband

2. Multitasking
   a. Covering two very sick patients
   b. Absence of a nurse's aide

3. Interruptions
   a. Pager constantly sounding
   b. Frequent changes in management plans for each patient

4. Low visibility labeling of the medication bags
   a. No policy for clear labeling of look-alike medication bags
   b. No labeling of intravenous tubing to allow a second check when hooking up the IV

c. No classification of or special handling procedures for dangerous drugs like norepinephrine

   d. No pharmacist to assist with administration of toxic drugs

After creating a list of primary and secondary drivers, what seemed at first glance to be a negligent act by the nurse in reality has multiple explanations, all of which focus on defective family and hospital systems. The nurse should receive classes on stress reduction and relaxation techniques to improve sleep. She and her family should also consider family counseling. All these interventions would reduce her fatigue and improve how she functions at work. By understanding the hospital system drivers, improvement teams can create process and structural improvements to correct the many dysfunctional hospital systems uncovered by this deadly error (see **Figure 3.6**).

Space does not allow a full description of the planning process; however, the specific methods that can be used to create reciprocally interdependent teams will be described in the next chapter. Effective working teams are capable of creating a rich catalogue of potential improvements (see right column in **Figure 3.6**). A carefully designed meeting agenda is critical for prioritizing discussion topics and decisions. These agendas should not be left up to a secretary but rather should be carefully created by the team leader with the input of other team members.

Do

Next, the preliminary operational changes and protocols planned in the conference room will need to be piloted in real-life situations and modified based on feedback from the frontline implementers. Therefore, for care protocols, decisions are never final; they are simply preliminary operational instructions. Given this reality, excessive deliberation may prove wasteful. Some quality experts recommend that quality teams devote no longer than twenty minutes to creating a new operating procedure to ensure that it is not overly complex. Experience has shown that overly complex operating procedures with multiple steps can actually increase errors or simply be ignored by frontline implementers[6]. These very busy care providers don't have the time to understand complex protocols and may instead work around them.

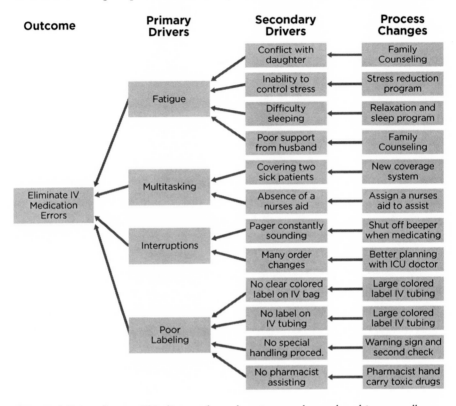

Figure 3.6. Driver diagram. This diagram shows the primary and secondary drivers as well as potential solutions for **Case 3.2A**.

The obvious first step improvements should be to label the medication bags with bright color-coded labels and to add a similar label to the intravenous tubing. Dangerous but therapeutically valuable and necessary drugs like norepinephrine should have a special danger symbol, perhaps a red exclamation point. In designing the label, the team needs to take into account the reactions of the patient and the patient's family. Just as for the RCA team, PDSA improvement teams will be far more effective if a patient or patient family member can be recruited to join the team.

Study

Daily medication error monitoring should begin prior to the intervention and continue after the improvement is initiated to ensure that a significant reduction in IV medication errors has been achieved.

Act

If a significant improvement is documented (i.e. if special cause variation is observed—see **Figure 3.2B**), then the new practices should be continued.

Repeat the PDSA Cycle (Figure 3.5)

At this point the team should carefully examine the new labeling process and plan other improvements. For example, they may now plan an educational program for caregivers to ensure that they understand and properly use the new labeling system. PDSA cycles should also be used to improve ICU nurse multitasking and to reduce interruptions. PDSA cycles are continued until the team is satisfied that they have addressed all of the most important primary and secondary drivers for the error and have decreased the intravenous medication error rate to zero. Meaningful improvement usually takes five to six PDSA cycles.

Failure Mode and Effects Analysis (FMEA)

Rather than waiting for an error to occur, medical safety experts have begun utilizing a practice commonly used in the aerospace, automotive, and airline industries called failure mode and effects analysis, or FMEA[6]. NASA used FMEA to successfully land a man on the moon, and this process helps to explain the remarkable safety record of the airline industry. This team-based process starts by identifying a high-risk process. Next the team fully describes the process to achieve a full understanding. Next they brainstorm to identify all the possible ways the system could break down, and they imagine the effects of each potential failure. Each failure is then prioritized based on the consequences or effects of the failure, and a proactive rather than a reactive root cause analysis is performed, followed by PDSA cycles to fix the process.

If FMEA had been performed to explore potential failures related to intravenous medication administration in the ICU before **Case 3.2A**, it is highly likely this potential error would have been included as part of the brainstorming session, listed as a high priority, and proactively fixed. FMEA could have prevented Mr. J.'s untimely death from a human error.

Forcing Functions

Given the reality of human error, one of the ideal strategies for improving reliability is to create systems that force the caregiver to always do the right thing. Anesthesiologists have led the way when it comes to designing forcing functions. In earlier times, a distracted anesthesiologist periodically hooked up a nitrous oxide source to an anesthesia machine in place of oxygen, with fatal consequences. For years those who made these errors were blamed and fired for negligence. Despite these punitive actions, the fatal error kept recurring. Eventually people realized that the gas administration system required continual attention and surveillance to ensure that the gas lines were correctly connected. This condition could be termed a latent error—that is, an error about to happen. Remembering the Deming's red bead experiment, this latent error could be classified as a red bead waiting to be discovered among the white beads.

Eventually the red bead was removed by redesigning the interlocking gas hose connectors. This new design created lock-and-key connections and only permitted the oxygen hose to connect to the oxygen tank and the nitrogen hose to connect to the nitrogen tank, forcing the anesthesiologist to always make the correct connection[14]. In addition, an oxygen analyzer with an activated audible alarm became a requirement for every anesthesia machine. Many hospitals employ human factors engineers whose purpose is to design equipment, systems, and working environments that minimize the likelihood of errors. If the intravenous tubing connectors for the norepinephrine had been designed so they could not be attached to the cefepime connectors, the ICU nurse would have been forced to match the right drug with the right medication pump.

Manual Checklists and Computerized Second Checks

Entire books have been written on the power of checklists[15], and given the complexity of modern medical care, no individual can possibly keep track of all the steps for a particular procedure in his or her working memory. Checklists provide a cognitive safety net that ensures that seemingly obvious steps integral to effective and safe care are not accidently overlooked[16]. Too often physicians complain that the use of checklists is cookbook medicine, and twenty-five years earlier, airline pilots raised similar concerns. However, checklists are now an integral element of the airline culture, and a pilot would never dream of beginning a flight without first running their checklist with the copilot.

Checklists combined with extensive training in systems, teamwork, and reliability have made the airline industry among the very safest industries in the world. And this industry has achieved six sigma; in other words the chances of a passenger being injured in an airliner crash are now less than 3.4 in a million. Although many of us are frightened during takeoff and landing, in reality we are far safer flying in a commercial airplane than crossing the street, driving a car, or being cared for in a hospital.

A major concern for nurses and physicians is the large number of procedures they are called upon to perform. Checklists need to be short, precise, and practical. An effective checklist should not exceed the capacity of our working memory and therefore should range from five to seven items. When a checklist exceeds nine to ten items, caregivers are likely to skip important items, defeating the purpose of reminding caregivers about critical steps in a care process. If a protocol requires additional steps, the checklist can be divided into subsections with five to seven items per subsection[16]. When it comes to experienced nurses, physician assistants, technicians, and physicians, do-confirm checklists are preferred. That is, the caregiver or team perform their jobs by memory or experience, and go through the checklist to confirm that no important step has been left out[16]. Checklists should serve as second checks rather than as so called read-do protocols that require the individual to check off each step as they do it. This is truly the cookbook approach that experienced caregivers complain about, and in most cases this approach should be avoided.

Checklists should be employed judiciously to avoid checklist fatigue. If caregivers are required to utilize excessive numbers of checklists, they are likely to ignore them. Another approach that serves the same purpose is to embed second checks within computerized ordering systems and in other automated machinery. Computer directed algorithms have great potential to ensure that the harried caregiver does not overlook important details.

Another effective tool that serves a similar role to checklists is the patient care bundle. A bundle is a grouping of evidence-based processes with proximate time and space characteristics that when performed collectively can improve outcome. Bundles have proven to be very effective for reducing ventilator-associated pneumonia (VAP), and the VAP bundle consists of five practices:

1. Head of bed elevation
2. Sedation vacation
3. Vein thrombosis prophylaxis
4. Peptic ulcer disease prophylaxis
5. Daily assessment of readiness to wean

In many intensive care units, when the VAP bundle is consistently applied, the rate of pneumonia has dropped to zero.

Similarly, the intravascular device bundle has proved to be very effective in reducing intravascular device infections and also consists of five practices[16]:

1. Hand washing
2. Use of full-barrier precautions with central line placement
3. Cleaning/prepping the insertion site with chlorhexidine
4. Avoiding the use of femoral catheters if possible
5. Removing all unnecessary catheters

As we discussed earlier, medication ordering, dispensing, and administering are the most common therapeutic processes in all hospitals, and computerizing these steps dramatically improves reliability[17]. The nurse in **Case 3.2A** was required by protocol to recheck the two medication bags upon returning from answering her page; however, in her rush to hang these important medications,

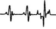

she inadvertently forgot her mandated visual second check. But what would have happened if all medication administrations were guided by barcodes?

Recently my wife, Kathie, and I were clothes shopping for our son Peter's birthday, and I noticed that the saleswoman in Macy's scanned a price tag barcode on each article of clothing we were purchasing. She next placed and scanned a second small barcode label over the price tag of each item to identify her as the person who had processed our purchase. I was impressed by the speed and ease with which she processed our sale. I realized there was virtually no chance for error. Barcode scanning allowed rapid identification of the item, its price, and the identity of the saleswoman. If this system had been in place in the ICU, the nurse could have scanned the norepinephrine bag and then scanned the medication pump setup to administer the antibiotic cefepime, and the scanner would have warned her that the medication bag and intravenous pump were incompatible. A barcode system in all likelihood would have saved Mr. J's life.

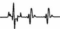

Key Points about Tools to Reduce Errors and Improve Reliability

- **RCA**—root cause analysis should be used to investigate all sentinel events (serious medical errors that cause death or serious injury or have the potential to do so, called near misses).
  - Perform within thirty days so memories don't spoil.
  - Recruit multidisciplinary team that includes a patient family member.
  - Identify all contributing factors and collect all data related to the problem.
  - Develop a quick fix followed by PDSA cycles.

- **PDSA Cycles**—plan-do-study-act cycles are a critical step in the process.
  - Ask three questions:
    - What are we trying to accomplish?
    - What change can I make that will result in improvement?
    - How will I know the change is an improvement?
  - Plan—develop an extensive understanding of the problem:
    - Use the five whys.
    - Construct a driver diagram exploring primary and secondary drivers.
    - Create as simple a change as possible.
  - Do—pilot the changes and modify based on frontline feedback
  - Study—utilize run and control charts to analyze performance measures.
  - Act—if the pilot represents an improvement, disseminate.
  - Begin the next PDSA cycle, and repeat at least four to five cycles to achieve continual improvement.

- **FMEA**—failure mode and effects analysis (FMEA) is used for potentially dangerous procedures.
  - Identify a high-risk process.
  - Brainstorm and imagine all possible ways the process could fail, and then prioritize.
  - Perform RCA, followed by PDSA cycles to proactively improve.

- **Forcing Functions**—create systems and equipment that forces the individual to always make the right choice.

- **Checklists and Second Checks**
  - Utilize do checklists.
  - Keep lists between five and seven items, never more nine to ten, or else break into subsections.
  - Utilize bundles for intravascular devices and ventilator-associated pneumonia.
  - Implement computer second checks for medication ordering.
  - Use barcodes to ensure accurate administration.

Second Victims

Case 3.2B. Mrs. J. was sitting by her husband's bedside. He was awake but required a respirator and breathing tube to maintain sufficient oxygen in his blood. The doctors were optimistic. He had a severe pneumonia; however, they told her he had no serious underlying diseases, and they predicted that after a few days of antibiotics he would improve and could be taken off the respirator. He was alert and frequently wrote short notes to let her know he was okay. Just before the nurse came in to hang the intravenous medications, he wrote, *I love you. Thanks for being here with me,* and he drew a little heart. Soon after the nurse administered the new medications, his eyes closed and his cardiac monitor began making ominous noises. The electrical cardiogram signal on the screen became irregular. A loud alarm sounded and "code blue, code blue" was paged overhead. Nurses and doctors rushed to her husband's bedside.

She watched the doctor pumping on his chest and was soon asked to leave the room. Twenty minutes passed as she sat with her eyes closed in the waiting room. The doctor came in with a sorrowful and guilty expression on his face. "There was nothing we could do. He had a cardiac arrest. His heart suddenly stopped pumping blood to the rest of his body. We lost him. I am very sorry." Mrs. J. stood up. She could not believe it. Mr. J. had looked so well, and then all of a sudden after the nurse started the new medications, he stopped responding to her. "Why did he suddenly die?" she asked the physician. He shrugged his shoulders and said, "We have no idea what went wrong. I am so sorry." He then quickly left the room, and the nurse came in several minutes later with Mr. J.'s belongings. She appeared very solemn and repeated over and over, "I am so sorry. I am so sorry."

At first, Mrs. J. was too shocked to cry. As she walked out of the hospital the reality sunk in; her husband of thirty-seven years would not be coming home. The tears poured down her face, and she crumbled to the floor of the hospital lobby. A guard rushed to her aid and escorted her to a chair. Over the next weeks and months, she heard nothing from the hospital or the doctors. When she inquired about the causes of her husband's death, she was greeted with a wall of silence. Anger and distrust combined with her sorrow made it very difficult for her continue her work at a local bank. Mr. J. was gone, and she suspected the doctors and nurses were at fault. She contacted a lawyer to investigate.

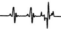

Mrs. J. is a second victim, and her suffering is impossible to comprehend. I know something of her profound sense of loss; however, unlike Mr. J., Mary managed to survive. Also Mary's progressive downhill course was caused by a series of smaller errors, while Mr. J. suffered a single very serious fatal error. His death came very suddenly and was unexpected.

Mr. and Mrs. J. represent a compilation of several cases that I have learned about through mortality and morbidity discussions, as well root cause analysis meetings, and they do not represent a single patient. You may ask why I couldn't include a real case. The major reason is fear of litigation. Sadly, the threat of malpractice suits has driven many of the improvement strategies so effectively used by other industries underground. I have participated in several root cause analysis meetings, and in each instance I have been instructed not to take notes for fear they would be "discovered." If a lawyer learns who attended an RCA, they can subpoena any notes taken by the participants. What this means is doctors can be punished for trying to understand what went wrong and trying to fix the problem.

It is no wonder so many nurses and doctors are afraid to speak to second victims like Mrs. J. However, there is a growing consensus based on interviews from victims of medical errors that silence breeds anger, distrust, and malpractice lawsuits. Many families want closure. They want to know what really happened to their family member. They also want to be assured that the hospital community will learn from their loved one's death and use that information to prevent others from dying of similar errors[18]. For these reasons, a complete explanation of the error, combined with empathy and a heartfelt apology, is strongly recommended. And in many cases family members should be encouraged to participate in the root cause analysis because they often provide helpful information. Furthermore, inclusion of a victim's family member assures everyone that everything is out in the open. Honesty and transparency are always the best policy.

The ICU nurse was also a second victim. Imagine her guilt and sorrow. Her goal as a nurse was to heal the sick and cure Mr. J. A simple error caused by multiple factors, many of which were out of her control, led to the death of her patient. Many caregivers who make such an error suffer deep depression, and many quit the medical field. Blaming the nurse and calling for her resignation, in my view, represents cruel and callous behavior, and this approach should be avoided except in cases of wanton negligence and disregard for patient welfare. She should instead receive counseling and emotional support. The ICU nurse was a victim of poor systems, and our goal should be not to blame her but to redirect our energy to improving our systems of care and preventing a similar medication error from ever reoccurring.

How the institution manages the ICU nurse who made the error in **Case 3.2A** sends a clear message to other caregivers. Counseling, education, and support rather than dismissal are the best course of action. In Mr. J.'s case, the system was primarily at fault and combined with the ICU nurse's high level of stress to promote a deadly error. Each case is unique, and although the majority of errors are caused by bad systems and not bad people, personal malfeasance and incompetence can also contribute to preventable injuries and death and require a more punitive approach.

How an institution responds to tragic mistakes tells caregivers, patients, and the community a great deal about the transparency, fairness, and sense of justice within an institution. How an institution responds during crisis greatly affects its climate of safety. Everyone aspires to work in a "good" institution— that is, an organization that is truthful and transparent and one that treats its patients and employees with dignity and fairness. The ideal response to Mr. J.'s death should have been to immediately acknowledge the mistake and to accompany this admission of guilt with a heartfelt apology to the family and the community. These actions should be followed by a public report to employees and the community explaining what went wrong and how the organization planned to fix it. The CEO should speak for the entire institution in expressing sincere regret and remorse, a sincere desire to learn from the mistake, and a strong commitment to continual improvement[18]. When these actions are accompanied by fair and just compensation of the victim's family, further legal action and expensive litigation can often be averted. But more importantly, such actions tell the community and the employees that their institution will do the "right" by its patients.

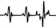

Key Points about Second Victims
- For the family left behind
  - closure and a full explanation are valued;
  - truthful and empathetic apology is the best policy;
  - full disclosure is the wisest course of action;
  - the threat of litigation often interferes with openness; and
  - full disclosure and demonstration of improvement to alleviate further errors reduces the likelihood of malpractice suits.

- For the caregiver who made the error,
  - they are often the victim of defective systems;
  - guilt and depression are the rule;
  - counseling and emotional support are usually the best course of action rather than punishment; and
  - their errors are usually the result of bad systems, not bad people.

- The leadership response to sentinel events tells patients, employees, and the community a great deal about the prevailing culture.

- "Good" institutions are just, fair, and open.

Public Reporting of Performance Measures

The Joint Commission, as well as many state legislatures, have mandated the public reporting of hospital-acquired infections including blood stream infections, urinary tract infections, ventilator associated pneumonia, and postoperative infections. Other reportable complications include pressure sores (called decubitus ulcers), falls in the hospital, performance measures for heart attack, and community-acquired pneumonia. Websites now rate overall hospital quality, as well as individual physician performances. Analysis of many of these websites remains difficult; however, Consumer Reports—renowned for its clear and objective ratings of automobiles, electronic goods, and household products—has begun to apply these methods to assess the quality of health care systems throughout the United States[19]. Before considering an

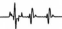

elective treatment or diagnostic procedure, patients will increasingly utilize the Internet to investigate the latest quality measures for their health care institutions. Nurses and physicians have a stake in improving these measures because the survival of their hospital system will increasingly depend on these quality measures.

Key Points about Public Reporting

- Public reporting of hospital acquired infections is now mandated.

- Performance measures for pneumonia and heart attack are also available on the Internet.

- Hospital quality is now being publically rated.

- Consumer Reports has a user-friendly evaluation system for comparing hospitals.

Conclusions

High-quality health care is safe as well as patient-centered and efficient. Safety depends on reliable systems, and at the present time most health care systems are highly unreliable with errors hovering between one per ten and one per one hundred. Industry aspires to fewer than three errors per million actions, and many have achieved this goal. In health care we have tremendous room for improvement. We must minimize conditions that increase human errors such as fatigue, stress, multitasking, and distraction. However, even more importantly, we must build systems that provide backups that correct for normal human errors. Vigilance and trying harder are not viable strategies and ignore the fact that "to err is human."

No matter how hard individual caregivers try, they will make mistakes. We must apply the tools for improving our systems of care: root cause analysis (RCA), plan-do-study-act cycles (PDSA), and failure mode and effect analysis (FMEA). We need to build in forcing functions that force caregivers to always do the right thing, and we need to use checklists and design second checks for our computer programs and equipment. Finally, we need to improve the climate of safety and create organizations that are transparent, just, and caring.

References

1. F. S. Southwick, and S. J. Spear. 2009. Commentary: "Who was caring for Mary?" revisited: a call for all academic physicians caring for patients to focus on systems and quality improvement. *Acad Med* 84 (12):1648-1650.

2. Gerald J. Langley. 2009. *The improvement guide : a practical approach to enhancing organizational performance. 1st ed, Jossey-Bass business & management series.* San Francisco: Jossey-Bass.

3. Michael E. Porter, and Elizabeth Olmsted Teisberg. 2006. *Redefining health care : creating value-based competition on results.* Boston, Mass.: Harvard Business School Press.

4. L. L. Leape. 1994. Error in medicine. *JAMA* 272 (23):1851-1857.

5. J. Reason. 2000. Human error: models and management. *BMJ* 320 (7237):768-770.

6. A. Frankel, M. Leonard, T. Simmonds, C. Haraden, and K.B. Vega. 2009. *The Essential Guide for Patient Safety Officers.* Oakbrook Terrace, IL: Joint Commission Resources, Inc.

7. A. M. Williamson, and A. M. Feyer. 2000. Moderate sleep deprivation produces impairments in cognitive and motor performance equivalent to legally prescribed levels of alcohol intoxication. *Occup Environ Med* 57 (10):649-655.

8. D. R. Gold, S. Rogacz, N. Bock, T. D. Tosteson, T. M. Baum, F. E. Speizer, and C. A. Czeisler. 1992. Rotating shift work, sleep, and accidents related to sleepiness in hospital nurses. *American journal of public health* 82 (7):1011-1014.

9. K. Graves, and D. Simmons. 2009. Reexamining fatigue: implications for nursing practice. *Critical care nursing quarterly* 32 (2):112-115.

10. L. D. Scott, A. E. Rogers, W. T. Hwang, and Y. Zhang. 2006. Effects of critical care nurses' work hours on vigilance and patients' safety. *American journal of critical care : an official publication, American Association of Critical-Care Nurses* 15 (1):30-37.

11. E. R. Stucky, T. R. Dresselhaus, A. Dollarhide, M. Shively, G. Maynard, S. Jain, T. Wolfson, M. B. Weinger, and T. Rutledge. 2009. Intern to attending: assessing stress among physicians. *Acad Med* 84 (2):251-257.

12. B.E. Trusko, C. Pexton, H.J. Harrington, and P. Gupta. 2007. *Improving Healthcare Quality and Cost with Six Sigma*. Upper Saddle River, N.J.: FT Press.

13. L. L. Leape. 2010. Personal Communication.

14. R.M. Wachter. 2008. *Understanding Patient Safety, Lange Series*. New York, NY: McGraw-Hill.

15. A. Guwande. 2009. *The Checklist Manifesto: How to Get Things Right*. New York, NY: Henry Hold and Company, LLC.

16. B. D. Winters, A. P. Gurses, H. Lehmann, J. B. Sexton, C. J. Rampersad, and P. J. Pronovost. 2009. Clinical review: checklists - translating evidence into practice. *Crit Care* 13 (6):210.

17. D. W. Bates, J. M. Teich, J. Lee, D. Seger, G. J. Kuperman, N. Ma'luf, D. Boyle, and L. Leape. 1999. The impact of computerized physician order entry on medication error prevention. *J Am Med Inform Assoc* 6 (4):313-321.

18. J. Conway, F. Federico, K. Stewart, and M.. Campbell. 2010. Respectful Management of Serious Clinical Adverse Events. . *IHI Innovation Series white paper.*, http://www.IHI.org.

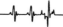

19. Consumers Union. [cited October 8, 2011]. Available from http://www. consumerreports.org/health/doctors-hospitals/hospital-ratings.htm.

Chapter 3 Exercises

1. What systems or system do you work within?

    a. Draw a diagram to show how your system works.

    b. Where do you fit into the system?

    c. Have you noticed dysfunctional parts of the system?

2. Recall recent errors you have made. What factors made your errors more likely?

3. Have you made a serious error that has caused you or others harm?

    a. Perform a root cause analysis.

    b. Create a series of PDSA cycles to improve this situation to prevent it from ever happening again.

    c. How would you measure the changes you propose to ensure they are improvements?

4. How does your institution respond to sentinel events?

    a. Does the administration encourage transparency?

    b. Does the institution blame individuals for errors?

    c. Do you feel your institution is a "good" institution?

-4-

Championship Teams Make No Excuses

How Could a Team Approach Have Improved Mary's Care?

Guiding Questions

1. What key conditions are required to create a successful team?

2. Why is team structure important? And what happens if you have too little or too much structure?

3. What does a "bounded" team mean?

4. What is meant by a team launch?

5. Are there resources that need to be provided to ensure that a team succeeds?

6. When and how should a team be coached?

7. How do you ensure that a team continues to improve?

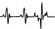

Lost Opportunities

Mary's illness was complex and required the input of general internists and specialists in cardiology, neurology, kidney disease, pulmonary disease, hematology (blood diseases), orthopedics, and infectious diseases. Her illness was also continually evolving, and these challenging conditions required efficient and seamless communication and coordination. There are very few individuals that would be capable of managing Mary's complex array of data, as well as the multiple viewpoints of seven subspecialists.

The physicians who first cared for Mary in the hospital were a working *group* and not a working *team*. They worked as individuals and failed to communicate or coordinate their efforts. The nurses were never included as part of their group, and despite their knowledge about the subtherapeutic heparin dosing, the steep power gradient prevented Mary's bedside nurses from sharing their knowledge. There was no evidence of interdependence in the group's working relationships. The inexperienced intern appeared to be working alone. Based on the absence of appropriate laboratory data on the flow sheets, and his underdosing of Mary's blood thinner, I assume that he had received little help or supervision from his senior resident, the attending physician, or the other intern on the team. These conditions suggested that Mary was strictly his responsibility and not the responsibility of the entire group. Furthermore, he never asked for help from the bedside nurses because to request help would be considered a sign of weakness and would have violated the strict hierarchy and prevailing belief that physicians were infallible and solely in charge.

The fact that the attending physician was unaware of the inappropriately low anticoagulation dosing indicates that the intern and senior resident, as well as the bedside nurses, were not communicating important clinical information about Mary's hospital progress. Furthermore, the "team" had failed to fully discuss the helpful input of the consultants or to create an integrated action plan. The attending physician admitted to me that he had delegated the responsibility of coordinating Mary's care to the senior resident; however,

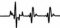

the senior resident either was unaware of the shift in responsibility or did not have sufficient expertise to accomplish this task. As a consequence, no new therapeutic interventions were begun or modified. This inaction allowed Mary's illness to progress from a modest number of clots in her legs to large blood clots that migrated to her lungs and then to a heart attack. It was only after I transferred her care to the intensive care unit that a team approach was applied, and the input of the various consultants was integrated, leading to her life-saving treatment and full recovery.

How Can Teams Help?

In the business world, the use of teams has become increasingly popular. As the complexity of the business has increased, many leaders have realized that no single person can fully interpret the multiple variables or analyze the streams of data required to effectively guide their organization. In business, misdirecting resources and failure to adapt to changes in the environment can quickly lead to loss of competitiveness and bankruptcy.

When employees work together in a true team, multiple perspectives are shared, and members are encouraged to think actively. Creativity increases, and the team is able to solve increasingly complex problems by utilizing a multidisciplinary approach. Members of high-functioning teams grow by the cross-pollination of ideas and develop new expertise that increases each member's value to the organization. The development of group expertise and the cross-training of team members insulate the institution from individual loss. Finally, highly functional teams are energizing, inspiring, and morale boosting.

The complexity of medicine has also progressively increased. With the advances in biomedical research, the number of diagnostic and therapeutic alternatives available to health care providers continues to increase at a rapid rate[1]. Recognizing that no individual can hope to manage the full breadth of this rapidly escalating knowledge base, health care providers have addressed these complexities by creating subspecialists that focus on narrower and narrower aspects of medicine. The consequence of this adaptation has been a progressive fragmentation of care for our patients.

The traditions of individualism and hierarchical power structures have inhibited physicians, nurses, pharmacists, case managers, and other support personnel from joining together to care for our patients. Lack of teamwork in medicine results in poor to absent coordination of care, gross inefficiencies and waste, and frequent errors that lead to unnecessary injuries and deaths[2].

Remembering that the health of our people hangs in the balance, every health care provider needs to understand what it means to be part of a team, how to work in a team, and how to lead a team. Just as physicians and nurses need to learn the fundamentals of taking a history and performing a physical exam, all health care providers need to fully understand the fundamentals of true teamwork.

Key Points about Why Teams Can Help

- Single leaders are unable to manage the increasing complexity:
  - Data and analytical challenges
  - Danger of misappropriating resources
  - Rapidly changing environment
  - Danger of business failure and bankruptcy

- Teams have many advantages:
  - Shared perspective
  - Multidisciplinary approach
  - Cross-pollination and growth
  - Protection of the institution from individual loss
  - Energy, inspiration, and improved morale

- Teams in medicine today are
  - blocked by individualism and hierarchical power structures and
  - a medical necessity; all health care providers must understand what it means to be part of a true team.

When Can Teams be Helpful in Medicine?

A team approach should be considered in medicine when the following elements are present[1]:

1. *Challenges to the traditional methods of operation*—The low quality and high error rate associated with today's medical care challenge our traditional methods. When old methods are no longer working, new methods should be designed and disseminated. Teams of experts can collaboratively solve problems and design new methods far more effectively than a single person. Furthermore, the involvement of caregivers and administrators from multiple disciplines creates commitment to a new way of operating and encourages meaningful change.

2. *Requirements for horizontal integration of semiautonomous individuals or units*—In medicine, physicians view themselves as semiautonomous. In addition, medical specialty departments, particularly in academic medical centers, view themselves as autonomous and in some cases compete with each other for resources.

   For example as health systems begin to focus on patient-centered product lines such as solid organ transplantation, the financial interests of the individual departments can interfere with the creation of these multidisciplinary services[3]. Historically, departments of surgery have received the bulk of the profits from transplantation and have used these profits to subsidize nontransplant surgeons performing less profitable procedures. If transplant services were to become independent financial and administrative entities, departments of surgery would lose this major profit stream. However, this change would be expected to motivate transplant teams to improve efficiency, reduce costs, and reduce charges to make their services more competitive.

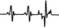
Furthermore, members of different departments often fail to respect each other's expertise and contributions. The consequences of these conditions are fragmented and error-prone care for our patients, and Mary is a prime example. Multidisciplinary teams promise to overcome these dysfunctional silos.

3. *Needs for information exchange to achieve alignment and coordination*— Many of the errors in medicine can be attributed to poor communication and a lack of information sharing[4]. Too often physicians fail to share their treatment plan with nurses or to discuss justifications for their decisions. In turn nurses are unable to clearly explain their treatment plan to the patients. Furthermore, when the nurse does not understand the treatment plan, he or she is unable to make any independent decisions and is required to repeatedly page the physician for clarification. This wastes time for both the nurses and the physicians.

4. *Complex decisions about critical issues*—In health care, decisions are too often made by a single individual. Such decisions are often poorly orchestrated and take place in the absence of a complete understanding of the issues or the application of accepted practices[5, 6]. No single person possesses the knowledge, perspective, or analytical skills to manage many of today's complex health care challenges.

There are multiple levels within health care where teams have the potential to be highly effective for improving our dysfunctional systems. Senior leadership teams at both the local and national level can be formed to address many of the high-level structural and administrative impediments that have slowed innovative change. Multidisciplinary teams can be assembled to coordinate the delivery of specific services such as solid organ transplantation, coronary artery disease, stroke, and acute gastrointestinal bleeding. Similar teams promise to be effective for coordinating other elective surgical procedures and for the management of many chronic medical disorders including diabetes mellitus, hypertension, congestive heart failure, arthritis, and AIDS.

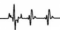

Every inpatient service must conduct work rounds daily on their hospitalized patients. Formation of true multidisciplinary rounding teams that include physicians, nurses, pharmacists, and case managers have the potential to improve patient flow and patient satisfaction, reduce errors, and improve caregiver job satisfaction[7]. As previously discussed, a multidisciplinary team would have provided multiple checks that would have quickly detected Mary's subtherapeutic heparin dosing.

In the outpatient arena, multidisciplinary teams, sometimes termed medical homes, can provide patients with comprehensive care in a single visit rather than requiring patients to run from appointment to appointment to see multiple specialists in different offices and on different days. Teams can be formed to address specific health care quality issues such as improving vaccination rates, preventing patient falls, reducing pressure ulcers, preventing ventilator-associated pneumonia, and reducing nosocomial infections.

Key Points about Deciding if You Need a Team
- Teams should be considered when there are
  - challenges to the traditional methods of operation;
  - requirements for horizontal integration of semiautonomous individuals such as physicians;
  - needs for information exchange to achieve alignment and coordination; and
  - complex decisions that need to be made about critical issues.

- Teams can be used in health care systems in
  - senior leadership teams;
  - multidisciplinary patient care teams both in and out of the hospital; and
  - health care quality and safety teams.

Case 4.1. As the senior physician attending on the general medical wards, I noticed that work rounds often lasted four hours, from 9:00 AM to 1:00 PM . The medical residents presented unnecessary details about their patients, and these presentations were often followed by long attending physician monologues. Furthermore, there was little communication with the bedside nurses, and as a consequence, nurses were required to repeatedly page the physicians during rounds. The excessive time required for work rounds was interfering with the admission of new patients and causing a backup of patients waiting to be admitted from the emergency room. The entry of new orders and the arrangement of discharges were also being delayed, impairing the ability of the nurses to care for their patients and delaying patient flow on the wards. To make matters even worse, the residency training director was complaining that the residents were missing the noon educational conference, and the director of nursing was complaining about delays and lack of clarity of the physicians' treatment orders. What could I do to improve these poorly functioning groups?

Creating Highly Functional Teams

In order to solve the problems described in **Case 4.1**, everyone working in medicine will need to have a thorough knowledge of the five key conditions that lead to effective teamwork. Highly functional teams require compelling goals, sufficient structure, a stable number of team members with the proper skills, the appropriate resources, and continual coaching (see **Figure 4.1**)[1]. When these conditions are established, teamwork progressively improves, and as described in the following sections, establishment of each of these conditions helped to improve how the rounding groups in **Case 4.1** functioned.

Purpose: Creating Measurable Goals that Inspire

The first and most important condition is to create compelling, meaningful, and measurable goals for your team. Team goals should have personal meaning to the members of your team, and they should also to be perceived as significantly advancing the institution's mission. Fortunately in health care systems, the overall mission—to improve the health of fellow human beings—has great personal meaning, and a large percentage of those who choose health care as a profession have a strong personal commitment to this goal.

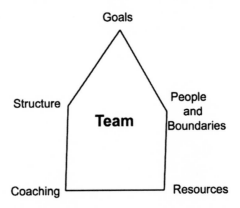

Figure 4.1. The five key conditions required for team effectiveness

When creating specific measurable goals for a team, it is important not only that the goals closely relate to the overall systems-wide mission, but that they also need to be compelling. One of the most effective ways to make health goals compelling is to link them to a specific patient, and we will discuss this strategy later. In addition to being inspirational and compelling, team goals must be achievable and measurable. The ability to measure progress provides feedback that allows the team to continuously improve their performance.

For example, as the senior physician on the rounding group in **Case 4.1**, I created a very specific and measurable goal: completing work rounds within two hours. In **Case 4.2**, the team chose to create policies for surgical antibiotic prophylaxis, preoperative screening for MRSA, diagnosis and treatment of ventilator associated pneumonia, adherence to hand washing, and antibiotic prescribing on the bone marrow transplant service. Each goal had a number subgoals creating excessive complexity, making assessment of true progress difficult, and overwhelming the team. When the goals are overly ambitious and overly complex, the team will become distracted and discouraged, and as occurred in **Case 4.2**, the team will eventually dissolve.

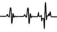
Case 4.2. As an infectious diseases consulting physician, I had noticed an increase in the number of patients infected with antibiotic resistant pathogens within our tertiary care hospital. I decided to organize a team to explore new ways to reduce these infections. In order to be politically correct, I invited the highest-ranking administrator from each discipline. I recruited the director of nursing infection control (who had served in this role for more than twenty-five years), the physician hospital epidemiologist, the director of clinical microbiology (who had served thirty years in this post), two head nurse supervisors, the head of pharmacy, an assistant pharmacist, two additional infectious disease experts, and a highly regarded surgeon (who had served thirty years), creating a total of eleven team members.

At our first meeting, the dean of the medical school personally charged the team to reduce infections and emphasized the importance of the committee for improving the quality of care. I next led a discussion concerning the goals of the team. As a group we came to a consensus on four goals that were complex, and that were not associated with clear measurable outcomes.

I failed to establish norms for behavior, and at the next meeting, the infection control nurse devoted the entire meeting to sharing her hospital infection data. The surgeon became upset about being unable to contribute his ideas and demanded the team use *Robert's Rules of Order* to assure a more orderly and balanced discussion. The hospital epidemiologist became frustrated because he felt that formal rules would inhibit his ability to share his ideas.

The team never gelled and failed to make significant progress. Attendance deteriorated, and I dissolved the team as a waste of everyone's time. I was disappointed and wondered if a team was a wise choice for solving these serious problems.

Key Points about Team Goals

Goals need to follow these guidelines:

- They must have personal meaning to team members in that they
  - should relate to patients and
  - need to be inspirational and compelling (touch the heart).

- They must be measurable to allow meaningful feedback.

- They must be developed with the team to ensure acceptance.

Team Structure: Creating Sufficient Structure to Enhance Team Function

Team structure is the second essential element for effective teamwork. Groups that fail to establish the proper structure do so at their own peril. What can happen if a supportive structure is absent? In the mid-1960s young people protesting the Vietnam War and the "establishment" abhorred structure and authority. The women's rights movement arose during this era, and as described by women's movement activist Jo Freeman in her classic article, these groups were renowned for their free flowing meetings that lacked all formal structure and leadership[7].

Women gathered in groups, shared their stories, and raised each other's consciousness. Participants took pride in avoiding "elitism" by eschewing any hierarchy or authority. Everyone was supposed to be equal. However, problems began to arise when these groups tried to work toward specific goals.

Without structure and leadership, no decisions could be made, and instead of an explicit leadership structure, implicit leaders subtly gained authority that was often based on prior friendships. Without appointed spokespersons and without structure or formal leadership, most of these women's groups failed to achieve significant progress and disbanded[7]. The women's movement learned from these mistakes and subsequently created highly effective teams that have facilitated the rapid advance of women's rights in many regions of the world[8].

What happens if there is excessive structure? The analysis of an international airline reveals the downside of too much structure. Based on market research, the airline created explicit protocols for all processes. Crewmembers were extensively trained, and each member was assigned a series of discrete tasks that they performed during the flight. To allow flexibility in scheduling, crewmembers were reassigned to a new team after each flight, and on average, individuals worked with the same crewmember once every five years.

Surveys indicated that service was reliable and overall customers were satisfied. The service provided was predictable and competent. However, employees failed to innovate, and ground-level improvements never occurred. All changes had to originate from the central office, and because of the complex procedural details, all changes required the rewriting of protocols and retraining of all flight attendants.

These processes were labor intensive and slow, explaining the airline's inability to keep up with their competitors' more innovative services. Crewmembers were hesitant to tailor their services to specific circumstances, having been taught that there was only one "best way" to provide each service. Often these specific routines worked for the typical flights but were not ideal for other situations. Flight attendants did not feel they had the right to modify the protocols despite realizing they were not ideal. By creating excessive structure, the airline underutilized the intelligence and creativity of its frontline workforce. For many employees, their job had little meaning and generated little excitement. It was "just a job"[9].

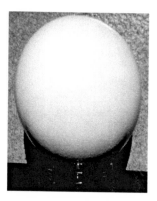

Figure 4.2. Team structure is analogous to an eggshell.

Team structure is analogous to an eggshell protecting the growing embryo[9] (see **Figure 4.2**). If the shell is too thin, it will break, killing the embryo. And the early women's rights movement exemplifies the consequences of insufficient structure. If the shell is too thick, the fully developed embryo will be unable to break out of its confining shell. And the highly structured protocol-driven international airline exemplifies the consequences of excessive structure. The ideal structure should provide a loose framework that is adaptable but has sufficient structure to foster true teamwork.

Key General Points about Team Structure

- Team structure is analogous to an eggshell:
  - Insufficient structure impairs team skill improvement and productivity.
    . Too thin an eggshell fails to protect the developing embryo.
  - Excessive structure disempowers and underutilizes the intelligence and creativity of the team members.
    . Too thick an eggshell prevents the embryo from hatching into a free living chick.

- Four components of an ideal structure are 1) meaningful jobs, 2) explicit team norms, 3) explicit governance and organizational structure, 4) the right number of people on the team.

Four tasks need to be completed to ensure a supportive team structure: 1) create meaningful jobs, 2) establish team norms, 3) create explicit governance, and 4) decide on how many members to have on the team.

1. Create Meaningful Jobs

To create jobs that are meaningful and internally motivating, ask five questions:

1. *Task identity*—is the task discrete in nature, and can one individual or one single group complete the task?

2. *Task significance*—does the task have a direct impact on the world, and is it clear how the task will assist in achieving the goals of the team?

3. *Skill variety*—does the task require the use of multiple skills?

4. *Autonomy*—will the task provide the freedom to make choices, adjustments, and improvements and allow the participant to learn by doing?

5. *Feedback*—will the results of the task be visible to the participant?

These individual characteristics can each be graded by an outside observer or job consultant from one (meaning never) to five (meaning always). A high score in task identity, task significance, and skill variety allows the team member to experience meaningfulness. A high score in autonomy encourages responsibility, and a high score in feedback encourages learning and increases knowledge. The most meaningful and internally motivating jobs will score a total of twenty-five. Whenever possible, tasks scoring in the five to fifteen ranges should be redesigned because such low-scoring tasks will reduce job satisfaction and motivation.

If these same principles are applied to the goals of the team as a whole, collective internal motivation can also be fostered. When teams are given full responsibility for completing their work, are assigned a broad variety of tasks that are discrete in nature, and are provided with timely performance measures, the collective motivation and team identity can be enhanced to create a winning team. However, when tasks are designed for groups rather than individuals, there is a potential risk. One or more members of the team may choose to slack off. This has been termed a motivational decrement, social loafing, or free-riding, and it is a danger in most groups[10]. One of the most effective ways of minimizing this tendency is to keep the size of the team small. This condition allows the team leader to more effectively monitor individual effort and to encourage collective internal motivation.

In medicine, too often jobs fail to fulfill one or more of the above criteria. For example, in many circumstances physicians give nurses little respect or latitude. Physicians expect each nurse to follow their orders exactly. With the exception of institutions that are encouraging improved doctor-nurse communication, physicians rarely discuss their patients' care with the nurses except when something goes wrong. In this environment, each time a physician speaks to a nurse, the conditioned first response is likely to be "What did I do wrong?"

Continual negative feedback puts nurses on the defensive and destroys any sense of psychological safety. The expectation of many physicians is that nurses should blindly follow their orders. But unquestioning obedience often leads to medical errors[13]. Nurses should feel comfortable about questioning orders that they do not understand or feel are incorrect. Improved autonomy increases the nurse's sense of responsibility and also renders their tasks more significant. To enhance job satisfaction and reduce nursing turnover, nurse administrators and physician leaders must encourage active nurse involvement.

Before redesigning my rounding group to address the problems described in **Case 4.1**, I decided to first observe how other attending physicians conducted work rounds. Through the lenses of job significance and motivation, I quickly realized that most of the nursing work assignments had low motivational quotients (see **Table 4.1**). In nearly all cases, nurses were expected to simply follow the orders of their attending physicians and never participated in decision making. Another major problem I discovered was the large amount of time nurses had to devote to filling out forms. This task had extremely low task significance and skill variety scores (see **Table 4.1**). Third, I found that because of the hectic nature of many inpatient services, the physicians almost never provided meaningful feedback to the nurses caring for their patients, which impaired the nurses' ability to actively learn. Based on these observations, I redesigned the nurses' job descriptions within our team to greatly improve their motivation quotients (see **Table 4.1**).

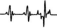

Table 4.1. Improving internal motivation of bedside nurses' work

Task	*Score TI/TS/ SV/A/F	Δ in Task	Score TI/TS/ SV/A/F
Standard work rounds: Attending makes all decisions, never asks the opinion of the bedside nurse, and only provides negative feedback	3/2/3/1/1 = 10	Encourage participation; act on nurse's ideas; encourage independent thinking and action; ensure frequent feedback	5/5/5/5/5 = 25
Filling out nursing forms	4/2/1/4/1 = 11	Have case manager assist with forms; create automatic electronic entry of vital signs	5/5/5/4/5 = 24
* TI = Task Identity, TS = Task Significance, SV = Skill Variety, A = Autonomy, F = Feedback			

A similar analysis and modification of tasks is warranted for all personnel within the health care system. Modifications of low-scoring tasks will increase job satisfaction and internal motivation throughout the system. These effects promise to improve morale and reduce personnel turnover.

Key Points about Creating Meaningful Jobs for Teams

- All jobs need to be designed to maximize internal motivation (max score of twenty-five):
  1. Task identity must be discrete (five points maximum for each).
  2. Task significance should be high.
  3. Skill variety should be high.
  4. Autonomy should be high, allowing task adjustment and creativity.
  5. Feedback must be rapid, accurate, and clear.

- Too often medical jobs have low internal motivation quotients (less than fifteen points).
  ○ Nurses

    - have minimal autonomy;
    - are expected to simply follow the doctors' orders without meaningful explanations; and
    - receive primarily negative feedback from physicians.

- All jobs in medicine need to be reexamined for internal motivation and redesigned when scores are low.

Case 4.3. Dr. D., a consulting physician, began screaming at the ICU bedside nurse just outside the door of a critically ill patient. Dr. D. was furious that a procedure to drain the fluid from the lung of his patient had not been performed. A medical resident rushed over to calm the situation but was loudly rebuked. Both the resident and nurse looked on as Dr. D. jumped up and down and, as described by another observer, acted like a two-year-old throwing a tantrum. As noted in the letter of complaint by the head floor nurse, Dr. D. demeaned his profession, upset the bedside nurse as well as fellow physicians, disturbed several families that were trying to cope with the imminent death of loved ones, and embarrassed everyone.

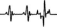

2. Establish Explicit Team Norms

Team leaders that assume behavioral norms will naturally evolve during team meetings need only to read **Case 4.2** to realize that without explicit norms, behavior can quickly deteriorate. One of the initial tasks of a new team should be to decide on a small number of things members should *always do* and *never do*. By establishing these explicit behavioral boundaries, team member anxiety can be reduced, and the freedom to fully express individual views is likely to be enhanced. A nearly universal *always do* should be to welcome and value the voice of every team member. For example, a multidisciplinary rounding team in nonemergency situations could agree to *always* allow the most junior members of the team to speak first to ensure that their ideas are heard before the more senior members of the team. Such an agreement would encourage true collaborative decision making rather than unilateral decision making by the senior physician.

Patient safety experts have recognized that the important "never" behavioral event described in **Case 4.3** quickly destroys morale and disrupts teamwork. Physicians, nurses, and health care providers should *never* be abusive and disrespectful. In their *Sentinel Event Alert* of July 2008 the Joint Commission stated: "Intimidating and disruptive behaviors can foster medical errors, contribute to poor patient satisfaction and to preventable adverse outcomes, increase the cost of care, and cause qualified clinicians, administrators, and managers to seek new positions in more professional environments"[12]. The Joint Commission noted that intimidating and disruptive behaviors include "overt actions such as verbal outbursts and physical threats, as well as passive activities such as refusing to perform assigned tasks or quietly exhibiting uncooperative attitudes during routine activities"[13]. These behaviors are unprofessional and should not be tolerated. As described in **Case 4.3**, such actions can be precipitated by delays in therapy, as well as by other manifestations of dysfunctional systems. The delay in lung drainage in **Case 4.3** occurred because the doctor responsible for performing this procedure was required to attend an outpatient clinic for the entire afternoon. He returned to the ward two hours after Dr. D.'s tantrum and successfully performed the procedure.

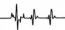

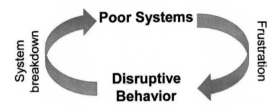

Figure 4.3. The downward spiral of disruptive behavior and dysfunctional systems

As shown in **Figure 4.3**, poorly functioning systems cause delays and errors that increase frustration. Frustration in turn can precipitate disruptive behavior that, as the name implies, disrupts the system by distracting caregivers, damaging interpersonal relationships, and breaking apart previously well-functioning teams. Disrupted systems create further frustration and increase the likelihood of further harmful emotional outbursts. Sadly, despite multiple policy papers and studies documenting the costs of disruptive behavior, many institutions have been reluctant to fully address this important issue. We all must understand that to "permit is to promote"[14].

GATEWAY

http://bit.ly/sZcBae

In addition to creating explicit behavior boundaries, each team should create other expectations to enhance teamwork. All team members should be as committed to their team as they are to their individual roles. A strong

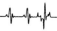

commitment to the team enhances team identity and team spirit. For example, when I observed other rounding groups, I noticed that residents with fewer patient assignments left the hospital early each day, leaving the other residents with larger numbers of assigned patients behind to complete their additional work.

To improve team function described in **Case 4.1**, I expressed the expectation that all members of my team should contribute equally to the workload of the team. This expectation encouraged the residents on my team to share their work and to leave the hospital together once all the work of the team had been completed. If the rotating ENT intern caring for Mary had been part of such a team, he would not have worried about being stigmatized by asking for help. Similarly floor-nursing teams should share their workloads and assist each other. When one nurse has difficult and labor-intensive patients, other members of the floor team should keep a vigilant eye on him or her and be ready to pitch in. Constant communication and an understanding that everyone sinks and swims as a team encourages everyone on the team to call for help when they are overwhelmed.

Once the behavioral norms have been established and agreed upon by the team, it is critical that all infractions of these norms be quickly addressed. Without timely and consistent enforcement by the entire team, team norms will be of no functional benefit.

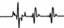

Key Points about Team Norms

- Behavioral norms need to be explicitly created by the team.
  - They should decide what team members will *always do*:
    - Everyone should always encourage participation by all team members
    - Everyone should value all team members opinions
  - They should decide what team members will *never do*:
    - Team members should never exhibit disruptive behavior (as designated in the Joint Commission's *Sentinel Event*) because it
      - increases medial errors and
      - destroys teamwork

- Commitment norms
  - They should demonstrate equal commitment to the team as to individual work.
    - Work should be shared among team members.

- Once the norms have been established, they need to be enforced quickly and consistently by the team.

3. Create an Explicit Team Governance and Organizational Structure

As noted in the earlier discussion of the early women's movement, lack of leadership prevents the achievement of meaningful team goals. To be effective, each team must have an explicit leadership structure. In some teams, leadership can be shared, while in others a single leader is most effective. In nearly all health care delivery teams, including surgical teams, inpatient rounding teams, and resuscitation teams, a single physician or nurse will need to be ultimately in charge to ensure timely and decisive action. However, declaring a single team leader carries with it the danger of creating a steep authority gradient or hierarchy. Many of the most disruptive and unprofessional behaviors have been observed in team leaders that have been given ultimate authority. Furthermore, steep authority gradients inhibit communication and reduce

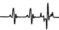

the sense of psychological safety among lower ranking team members. Team leaders should try to reduce this power gradient by encouraging humility and by actively encouraging others to contribute their ideas.

Those who are familiar with medicine and surgery are likely to believe that the team leadership structure is well understood and does not need to be explicitly described. However, failure to explicitly discuss who is in charge and why they have ultimate responsibility can lead to confusion about who is leading the team. If the reporting structure has not been clearly delineated, senior physicians may inadvertently abdicate their authority, leaving decision authority to less experienced residents in training. In other situations, a nurse may be the most appropriate person to lead a multidisciplinary team. Unless this is clearly spelled out, the nurse leader may be fearful or hesitant to take charge. In twenty-first century medicine, shared leadership is an important condition for improving the quality and safety of patient care.

Given the fact that many supervising faculty are required to multitask, as was the case for Mary's first inpatient medical attending physician, the resident may assume that the attending does not want to be "bothered" about patient management issues except during the specific times allotted for inpatient rounds. This approach withholds from patients the expertise of the most experienced physician on the management team—a condition that can result in errors, misjudgments, and permanent harm. Nurses on multidisciplinary rounding teams need to be aware of the issue, and I recommend they address such concerns with the attending physician. Mary's first inpatient attending was unaware of her subtherapeutic anticoagulation values and was caught off guard when I raised this issue after Mary suffered from blood clots to her lungs. If her nurse had requested that the senior attending be present at the bedside and actively intervene, I believe many of Mary's complications could have been averted.

As the senior attending physician in **Case 4.1** I explicitly stated to my new team that I was the ultimate authority because nurses, patients, and insurance companies expected that the most experienced physician would have the final say regarding management decisions. I also encouraged a flattening of the authority gradient by stating that I did not have all the answers and looked forward to soliciting the input of everyone on the team, including bedside nurses. I emphasized the importance of sharing ideas and of creating a nonjudgmental atmosphere where everyone could feel comfortable to contribute suggestions for improving patient care.

When rounding, all caregivers should also try to model ideal professional behavior, including being polite and considerate when interacting with team members and patients. I have always aspired to these goals, but I must confess that in the heat of battle, I, like many of my colleagues, do occasionally lose patience. Over my thirty years on the wards, I have come to realize the great value of self-control.

Team leaders are most effective when they serve as discussion leaders, and I embraced this role in my rounding team improvement project. By using the Socratic method consisting of guiding questions, I encouraged active discussions. I then summarized the deliberations of the team and arbitrated a final action plan when there was controversy. This approach allowed all members of my team to develop a sense of control over their work and improved their sense of autonomy.

Another key structural condition is the creation of a team agenda to ensure that the team focuses on their major tasks. Many teams inadvertently spin their wheels by focusing on trivial issues rather than asking the key questions and focusing on the major tasks. As described in **Case 4.1**, many rounding medical teams spend excessive time discussing irrelevant past history, normal physical findings, and normal laboratory values rather than focusing on the specific clinical details related to the patient's current illness. This inefficient approach wastes valuable time and often delays the ordering of the proper diagnostic tests and treatments.

As the senior attending physician, I insisted on succinct presentations that provided value-added information. I also suggested that the team designate specific time allocations for each patient, tailored to the complexity of each patient's active medical problems. By helping to prioritize the most active and

serious medical problems, I ensured that the team first focused on their patients'
most life-threatening issues.

Key Points about Team Governance and Organizational Structure
- An explicit leadership structure is required for productive teams.

- A single leader with ultimate authority is the rule for health care
  delivery teams.
  - Danger of authority abuse and higher risk of disruptive behavior
  - A steep hierarchy
    - Prevents formation of a zone of psychological safety
    - Inhibits free and open communication
    - Increases the risk of errors
    - Lowers job autonomy and internal motivation for other
      team members

  - Critical to flatten the authority gradient and develop a more
    horizontal power structure:
    - The leader must explicitly state the expectation that all members
      contribute to management decisions.
    - The leader must be polite and considerate.
    - The leader should lead by open-ended questions and the
      Socratic method.
    - The leader should serve as a discussion leader and final arbiter.
    - The leader should encourage job autonomy.

- The leader should create a team agenda based on input from
  the team members.
  - The agenda should be carefully designed to ensure that time is
    efficiently allocated.
  - Establish priorities.
  - Encourage succinct and value-added communication.

---

4. Decide on the Ideal Number of Team Members.

Intuition may suggest that the larger the team, the more productive it will be. However in reality, as teams get larger there are significant process losses including motivation decrement and coordination difficulties (see **Figure 4.4**). These process losses reduce productivity, and when teams reach a certain size, the process losses outweigh the incremental increase in resources represented by the addition of a new member[10]. Mary's first inpatient attending assumed that requesting additional subspecialist consultants would improve her care. However, as predicted by those who have studied teams, the large number of consultants interfered with coordination and paralyzed the decision-making process. Only after the responsibility for care was switched to the cardiologist was this logjam of expert opinions relieved and appropriate life-saving therapy begun.

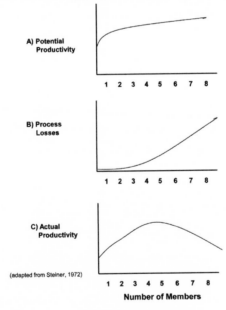

Figure 4.4. The effects of team size on process and productivity

In general, for decision-making teams, the ideal number should be six to seven, remembering that a six-member team consists of fifteen different pairs and a seven-member team consists of twenty-one:

$n \times (n-1) \div 2 = number\ of\ pairs$ (*n* is the number of team members)

As a general principle, the smaller the team, the higher the productivity per individual member. Larger teams can be assembled for alignment and informational teams where the primary purpose is the sharing of information. However, when it comes to productive, decision-making teams, smaller is truly better.

Key Points about Team Number
- Larger numbers of experts increase resources but cause process losses:
  - Resource gain must be balanced by process loss.
  - Coordination becomes more difficult.
  - Motivational decrement (social loafing) increases.

Boundaries and Stability: The Importance of Creating a Distinct Team that is Given Time to Progressively Improve

The team described in **Case 4.2** had members from multiple departments and disciplines. Rather than declaring a single member of the each department as a permanent team member, I allowed representatives to switch. I wrongly assumed that members from the same discipline and department were interchangeable. Each time a new member joined the team for a meeting, the other members had to review previous deliberations. As a consequence, the beginning of each meeting was devoted to bringing new members up to speed. Furthermore, new members often suggested new ideas related to old problems, requiring the team to revisit solutions that had already been agreed upon.

Case 4.2 exemplifies the importance of creating distinct boundaries regarding who is on the team and who is not. Unbounded teams are unlikely to develop consistent norms or a true team identity. For teams expected to make decisions and to coordinate operations, a stable roster is required. However, boundaries that are too strict can lead to isolation and a loss of perspective regarding the overall institutional goals. From time to time, outside experts will need to become temporary participants to solve specific

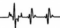

problems. In order to achieve some porosity and simultaneously maintain team identity, a core team that attends every meeting should be defined. When additional expertise or an outside perspective is required, temporary members can be invited with the understanding that they will attend team meetings for a defined period or until a specific problem is solved.

Once team membership has been defined, the core team should be given sufficient time to learn how to work together. It takes time to become comfortable with teammates and for each member to fully assess the strengths and weaknesses of other team members. And it takes time for the team to create and enforce their norms of behavior, learn how to effectively communicate, and develop a true team identity.

Data from commercial airlines bears on this important condition. The National Transportation Safety Board found that 73 percent of reported errors on commercial airline flights occurred on the crew's first day flying together[15]. The most dangerous time to be flying on a plane is the flight crew's first trip, when they are adapting to each other's individual styles and skills.

This finding raises concerns about common scheduling practices for both residents and nurses. To conform to the strict duty hour rules, many programs schedule frequent switches of residents within the inpatient rounding teams. Similarly, some nursing programs frequently insert temporary outside nurses to manage increased clinical demands in order to reduce their permanent staffing budget. Such frequent changes in team membership impair team function and would be expected to increase the likelihood of medical errors.

Utilizing flight simulation exercises, NASA has found that fatigued flight teams that had worked together for multiple shifts made significantly fewer errors than newly formed flight teams that were well rested[9]. Therefore as the research has verified, when it comes to error-free performance, *team stability can trump team fatigue.*

Many believe that team function deteriorates over time because team members become too familiar with each other and become lax in enforcing norms and following standard protocols[17]. They intuitively predict that within a short time of being together, performance will plateau. Based on these misunderstandings, many administrators believe that it is preferable to maintain a constant exchange of team members to prevent performance deterioration. However, **Case 4.4** and extensive research using objective measurements of team performance reveal the opposite outcome. The longer a team can be kept together, the better its performance and the closer the teammates become. Well-constructed teams continue to improve indefinitely[9].

> **Case 4.4.** Gale Danek was a student at the University of Michigan when she met a group of very politically active nursing students. She began attending health fairs that they were organizing and realized the exciting impact that team nursing could have on people's health. Upon earning a master's degree as a nursing clinical specialist, she joined a highly effective interdisciplinary team consisting of pediatric physicians and nurses. She served as an integral member of this care team for six years, later moving to a higher administrative role. However, to this day she remembers fondly the close camaraderie that developed among her team members and regards the many children whose lives she improved to be among her most meaningful accomplishments. She continues to regard her former teammates as close friends and continues to see them socially.

Key Points about Team Boundaries and Stability
- The team needs to have distinct boundaries:
  - o Everyone needs to know who is on the team and off the team.
  - o A core membership can be formed and allow temporary membership to provide temporary expertise.
  - o Without boundaries, norms and team identity cannot develop, and productivity will suffer.

- The team should be given sufficient time to learn to work together. It takes time to
  - o understand the strengths and weakness of teammates;
  - o effectively communicate;
  - o learn how to enforce norms; and
  - o develop team identity and team spirit.

- A fatigued team that has worked together produces fewer errors than a newly formed rested team. Team stability trumps team fatigue.

- Teams function better and better the longer they are together.

Creating a Supportive Organizational Environment: Recognizing Great Teamwork and Providing Team Resources

A new work team is like a young sprouting plant. It is delicate and requires nurturing conditions to grow and blossom. Too often administrators empower the formation of a team and then step away, assuming the team can fend for itself. However, without the proper organizational support, a team is unlikely to prosper and succeed. Teams require four key supportive resources: rewards, information, education[9], and administrative backup.

Rewards

Teamwork is associated with a potentially destructive inherent conflict. Team members are asked to devote valuable time to the team that could be devoted to their individual advancement within their organization. In many institutions, individual achievement is exclusively evaluated and rewarded. If this reward system remains in place, motivation to focus on individual personal projects will predominate and limit motivation to work on team projects. As an example, the University of Florida physician bonus program for the past five years has rewarded physicians who exceed their annual work target. Such targets reflect the physician's individual billing activity, and individual work volume has been the only metric for clinical reward.

If health systems truly want to foster teamwork, they must devote monetary funds and/or special recognition to reward team leaders and team members who participate in high-performing clinical teams. For such a reward program to be effective, team members must understand the performance metrics. Furthermore, these metrics must be directly affected by the team's collective behavior and must be accurately measured. Finally, team rewards must be contingent on achieving a superior performance score. For example, if administrators could identify quality care metrics such as length of stay, readmission rates, and appropriate timing of antibiotics for pneumonia and utilize these measures in addition to patient volume to reward care providers, this new reward system has the potential to motivate nurses and physicians to improve team performance in order to improve quality.

To improve and reward teamwork for my rounding improvement program, I decided to award all members of the team the same evaluation grade. And that grade reflected the performance and achievements of the rounding team. By working effectively together, the team members could and did earn an *A* (see **Case 4.1B** at the end of this chapter).

Information

As described earlier, one of the five determinants of job satisfaction is feedback. This important condition applies not only to individuals but also to teams. Without timely feedback, learning is compromised, and the team will be unable to appropriately adapt and improve. Feedback in health care means timely performance data.

Strategies for measurement and data management are critical for guiding any health care team. In many situations there is excessive data, and deciding which information relates directly to the team's specific goals is critical. Too often teams become excessively focused on data that has minimal relevance to their goals, resulting in wasted time and effort. If the key measures are not identified, the team is flying blind. Without the appropriate performance data, there can be no milestones, and the team will be unable to determine if they achieved their goals. To assess the progress of our rounding program (**Case 4.1**), I used the duration of work rounds as a very clear measure of performance and plotted a graph showing the duration of rounds each day, as well as the number of patients on our service (see **Figure 4.5**). This data motivated the team to maintain their efficiency on rounds, and as our team became more proficient, we consistently achieved our goal of rounding in less than two hours each day, despite a heavy clinical load. Later we also obtained length of stay and thirty-day readmission data (see **Figure 3.4**); however, these measures were calculated a month after we completed rounds and could not be used as feedback to guide our performance.

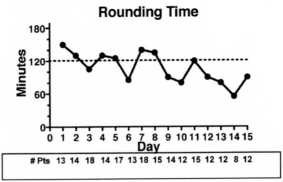

Figure 4.5. Time required to complete daily work rounds. Numbers on the bottom indicate the number of patients being managed by the team each day.

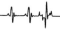

Education

Health systems have extensive training programs to ensure their employees have up-to-date skills, and the majority of training sessions are directed toward individuals. The training of a health care team as a unit is a less common practice. In the business community, training sessions for teams have become increasingly popular because these sessions have the potential to synergistically improve performance. Team members with differing expertise and perspectives share their learning with each other. The verbal processing of new information creates a very active learning environment that can enhance understanding, problem-solving capability, and long-term retention of facts. In recognition of this reality, many business schools are encouraging the formation of learning teams. For our rounding team, I provided handouts describing the basic principles of teamwork, and we learned together how to create an effective team. Medical schools and other health professional schools are beginning to adopt team-based learning (TBL). This teaching approach utilizes all of the principles described in this chapter and can experientially teach teamwork[18]. In May 2011, the national organizations representing U.S. nursing, physician, pharmacist, dentist, and public health colleges recommended that interdisciplinary education in teamwork and team-based care be required for all of their students[19].

Administrative Backup

Modern health systems have extremely complex structures that can be difficult to navigate. There are minefields everywhere, consisting of silos with rigid operating procedures that can impede team progress or, even worse, prevent the team from achieving its goals. These impediments can lead to frustration and quickly destroy team morale. Without a senior administrator with the proper authority to run interference, significant change and improvement may prove impossible, and the team's well-meaning efforts are wasted.

The inertia of the status quo cannot be overemphasized, and the importance of a senior administrator to serve as a minesweeper that removes these destructive roadblocks is in my view the single most important resource for bringing about change. Without strong and continuous support by administration, frontline improvements within our health care system promise to be exceedingly slow or nonexistent.

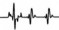

Case 4.5. I recently launched an eight-member quality improvement team consisting of two physicians, one nurse practitioner, four nurses, and a pharmacist. For the launch we followed the eight steps shown in **Figure 4.6**. Everyone introduced him or herself and described both their strengths and weaknesses. Together we discussed the goal of reducing the orthopedic postoperative infection rate. Next we decided on specific roles. One nurse agreed to serve as chairperson, and I agreed to serve as the secretary. Next we discussed the importance of a flat power gradient and the importance of everyone sharing their ideas. "Every idea is a good idea." Next we decided on our milestones: a reduction of postoperative infections from 0.45 percent to 0.10 percent over twelve months, with a 0.2 percent reduction at six months. Next we agreed on the behavior norms, including active involvement and ownership by those working on the front lines, mutual respect, and consistent attendance at every meeting. The team agreed that after a full discussion of each issue, the senior orthopedic surgeon on the team would serve as the final arbiter. Finally, to further motivate the team, I showed the YouTube video of Ginny, the patient who suffered a severe MRSA bone infection that led to amputation of her leg (see Chapter 6 for a full discussion of Ginny's story).

Launching a Team

How the team leader sets the stage for a newly formed team is a critical determinant of a team's future success. As the informal team leader in **Case 4.5**, I successfully launched our team, and as a consequence the team was highly motivated and had a strong likelihood of achieving its goal. Investigations of airline industry cockpit crews reveal that team dynamics and the likelihood of forming a highly functional team are determined within minutes by the airline captain's initial briefing[20, 21]. Crews that received any briefing by the captain did better than crews that received no briefing. Crews in which the captain espoused the positive features of the team, engaged the crew in a discussion about the unique circumstances of the trip, and created a structural shell proved to be the most competent and

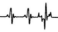

highly motivated.

What should ideally be accomplished during the launch? As shown in **Figure 4.6**, the first task is for the team members to begin to learn about each other. During introductions, each member should share the unique expertise and perspective he or she brings to the group. In addition, each member should share any weaknesses and any concerns about the team. By sharing personal details, team members can begin to establish trust and openness from the very beginning, as occurred in **Case 4.5**.

Team Launch

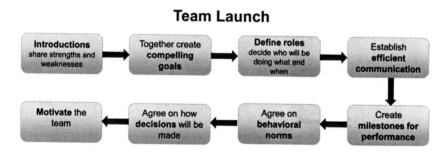

Adapted from Rosabeth Moss Kanter, Teamwork Toolkit, Harvard Business School, 2010

Figure 4.6 The eight steps for an effective team launch.

Upon completion of introductions, the person who convened the team can describe why the team was formed and explain in broad strokes what accomplishments are expected of the team. The introduction will launch a discussion of the team's mission and specific goals. In most cases, the team should come to a consensus about their mission and goals, as quickly occurred in **Case 4.5**. These two tasks should not be rushed and may take several hours or even several days depending on the complexity of the team's mission and goals. To accelerate this process, the convener can provide the team with introductory information several days prior to the meeting to allow team members to formulate preliminary ideas prior to the meeting. In **Case 4.5**, this process was accelerated by written documents that provided background information, allowing team members to quickly come to consensus on their measurable goal.

Once the team's goal or goals have been defined, the actual roles and responsibilities of each team member need to be agreed upon. Too often the team leader and the team members assume everyone knows their roles. However, without explicitly discussing this important issue, ambiguity prevails, and efforts will either be duplicated or certain tasks will be overlooked[22]. In **Case 4.1**, to achieve my medical rounding team launch, I invited the team members to lunch one week before the start of our rotation together. After introducing ourselves and agreeing on our goals, we as a group agreed upon the specific roles of the team resident: to distribute the workload evenly among the interns and medical students, organize discharges, contribute to all management decisions, set the agenda for morning rounds, and closely communicate with me as the attending physician. Similarly, the roles of other team members were discussed and agreed upon.

GATEWAY

http://bit.ly/tLwOK5

Particularly in medicine, the next critical step is to agree on how information will be communicated. In **Case 4.5**, in addition to face-to-face meetings, the team agreed to utilize group email. In **Case 4.1**, to ensure effective work rounds, the rounding team agreed that oral presentations should be succinct. Because electronic records were available, everyone agreed to read about the new cases before rounds, allowing the presenter to save time by summarizing key historical and physical findings, important laboratory findings, proposed diagnosis, and management plans.

Approximate deadlines for completion of each project should be established, and milestones should be created that delineate when each specific task should be completed. This provides the team with the motivation to act rather than simply discuss. The completion of milestones also gives the team a sense of progress and accomplishment. In **Case 4.5**, we agreed to a 0.2 percent decrease

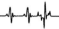

in postoperative infections within six months. In **Case 4.1**, the team agreed that we would involve all bedside nurses in our work rounds and spend a high percentage of our time interacting with our patients rather than talking in the hallways. These goals were measured by activity charts prepared each week by an industrial engineering intern. Finally, we agreed to complete rounds in less than two hours each day and plotted our rounding time at the end of rounds each day. Within several days, our team was consistently rounding in less than two hours (see **Figure 4.5**).

Once roles, communication protocols, and time lines have been created, team behavioral norms need to be established. Norms vary from institution to institution, as well as from department to department. For example, personnel in some departments or organizations may be comfortable with friendly teasing and interrupting, while other organizations may frown upon such behaviors. In **Case 4.2**, individuals from different departments had different expectations concerning communication styles. The surgeon preferred a formal style and wished to use *Robert's Rules of Order* for all discussions, while the hospital epidemiologist preferred a more free-flowing discussion that allowed interruptions. This team failed to discuss behavioral norms at the launch of the team, and these subsequent disagreements proved to be a source of persistent conflict.

When nurses actively participate on multidisciplinary rounds, they often have different expectations for behavior than physicians. Unless properly empowered, nurses tend to be less assertive than physicians, and their important viewpoints may be overlooked[11]. When team members from different departments with different ways of communicating are brought together, these differences need to be openly discussed and compromises regarding norms negotiated.

After agreeing upon behavioral norms, the team should next come to an agreement on how future decisions will be made. Too often teams prefer consensus; however, when team members are diverse in their viewpoints, consensus may prove to be very time consuming if not impossible to achieve. For medical teams whose primary mission is direct patient care, consensus may be sought; however, the final arbiter will usually be the senior attending physician or senior nurse leader. In **Case 4.5**, our team agreed that the senior orthopedic surgeon on the team would serve as final arbiter. In teams whose tasks are to develop new policies and operating procedures, a simple majority is often the most efficient approach. However, when there are one or more members who strongly disagree, the issue may need to be revisited.

Key Points about the Team Launch

- How the leader sets the stage is a key determinant for how well a team functions.

- An ordered launch increases the likelihood of success:
  - Allow the team members to
    - introduce themselves;
    - describe their expertise;
    - discuss weaknesses (increases trust); and
    - include any concerns about the team.
  - Provide a background regarding what motivated the formation of the team, followed by a discussion of the team's mission and goals.
    - The team needs to come to consensus about mission and goals.
    - Do not rush this step; the team must feel the goals are compelling.
  - Define the explicit roles and responsibilities of all team members to ensure there is no overlap and no missing roles.
  - Establish agreed-upon communication protocols for efficiency.
  - Create a carefully constructed agenda and agree on milestones, as well as the date for completion of the overall project.
  - Agree on behavioral norms.
  - Agree on the method for making decisions: 1) team leader has the final decision, 2) consensus, 3) simple majority.
  - Encourage interdependence and active sharing.
  - Arouse motivations to work for the team and to accomplish the team's goals.

The final elements of an effective launch are to motivate the team and to emphasize the importance of interdependence. The team leader should create a vision of how the sharing of the expertise by the group can achieve the team's goals. By emphasizing the importance of active sharing, the team leader begins to build a sense of team. The assigned work of the team needs to be placed into context, and the significance of the goals should be clarified by the end of the meeting. Just as an athletic coach arouses emotions and inspires the team before it takes the field, at the end of the launch the team leader can create a strong desire for team members to contribute their individual expertise and effort to the team's pursuit of success. In **Case 4.1**, I motivated my team by describing the ideal outcome: a highly efficient team that would allow the residents on average to leave the hospital two hours earlier than residents on conventional teams and at the same time provide the best possible care for our patients. In **Case 4.5**, a motivational video proved to be an effective motivator.

Managing Team Dynamics: When and How Should a Team be Coached?

In the ideal team, members openly share ideas and feed off each other as they create solutions to achieve their goals (reciprocal interdependence). Everyone feels safe to contribute ideas, and all members devote significant effort to achieving the team's goals. The expertise of each team member is utilized, and when one person disagrees with the group, the other members seriously consider the dissenter's point of view, as evidenced by reflective questions. The team achieves each milestone ahead of schedule, and as a consequence, team spirit is high. The team members are rewarded with compliments by the head of their department and also receive tickets to a popular Broadway play.

This ideal is difficult to achieve, and even the best teams encounter problems from time to time. There are many reasons why teams get off track. One of the most common problems has been termed *groupthink*. Team members develop the implicit norm that team harmony should always be preserved. When this norm develops, members feel uncomfortable expressing reservations about specific policies, and important dissenting viewpoints will not be expressed. The problem with this is that when the pros and cons of each idea are not fully explored, inappropriate policies or actual errors become

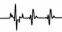

more likely.

All team members must be reminded that when groups come together for a shared purpose, conflict and anxiety are to be expected and can never be eliminated. Team members must learn to accept interpersonal tensions because the absence of tension and conflict indicates the members are no longer actively involved, and the working team has become a working group. Ideally the team should foster creative abrasion[23]. This condition occurs when the team members have diverse viewpoints, challenge each other, and welcome differences of opinion. Conflict must focus on ideas and avoid becoming personal in order to be perceived as constructive.

When open debate is encouraged, the range of information becomes broader, the understanding of issues deeper, and the possible solutions richer. The combination of multiple viewpoints creates a "kaleidoscope of ideas"[1]. One effective way of encouraging creative abrasion is to designate one team member as the devil's advocate. Their assignment is to generate opposing ideas. To have effective creative abrasion, team members need to be skilled debaters and/or have well formed, secure egos (i.e., thick skins).

A second threat to teamwork that is particularly common among medical teams is the tendency of team leaders to dictate team behavior. Often senior physicians prefer the spoked-wheel model of team leadership (see **Figure 5.1**). This leadership model creates a steep hierarchy of power, and research shows that under these conditions, those of lower rank are fearful of suggesting alternative solutions or of contradicting the conclusions of the leader, even when they know the leader is wrong[24]. One way to create a more horizontal structure is to insist that everyone call each other by their first name. Second, as described earlier during the team launch, the team leader should emphasize that he/she does not have a monopoly on ideas and, just like all humans, can make errors[25].

GATEWAY

ENTER

SIX

http://bit.ly/uKptmi

Key Points about Harmful Team Dynamics
- Groupthink
  - Describes the mistaken assumption that team harmony should be preserved
  - Results in the loss of dissenting viewpoints
  - Increases the risk of errors and inappropriate decisions

- Effective teams recognize that
  - Interpersonal tension is the normal state of all working teams
  - Promotion of creative abrasion enhances productivity
    - Encourages active discussion, airing of all viewpoints:
      - Criticize the ideas, not the person.
      - Assign a devil's advocate.

- A team leader who dictates team member behavior
  - creates a steep hierarchy;
  - discourages communication and increases errors.

- Hierarchy can be reduced by
  - calling everyone by their first name
  - acknowledging fallibility ("to err is human").

Coaching

What Behaviors Need to be Coached?

Because of time constraints, as well as the complexity of many of the tasks performed by medical teams, the team leader may not have the energy or time to stand back periodically and assess team dynamics. All teams need coaching, and in most circumstances an outside coach should be assigned to observe the team from time to time. Coaches can be peers or in some instances outside professionals with expertise in teamwork. Coaches should to focus on three elements:

1. *Effort*—how much effort are the individual team members expending to further the goals of the team? When there is social loafing, a redesign of tasks may need to be considered in order to increase intrinsic motivation (see the discussion on job significance above). The team leader and/or coach needs to quickly address social loafing because this behavior is one of the most common and serious forms of process loss. When the motivational gradient is unequal among team members, motivational issues can become the primary focus of the team, detracting from the overall productivity of the team. Ideally, when all members are highly committed to the team and are willing to contribute beyond expectations to improve team performance, there can be process gains. Team progress will be greater than predicted from the sum of the individual efforts. These higher performing teams are said to have great "team spirit" and a "can-do" attitude. They also demonstrate greater resilience, being capable of withstanding and overcoming greater challenges. Health care rounding teams usually have specific patient assignments and tasks and these conditions minimize the risk of loafing.

2. *Performance strategy*—in my experience, medical teams too often prefer traditional strategies and fail to incorporate innovative and time-saving approaches into their daily routines. Similar behavior is also commonly observed in business teams. Team members suffer from a paradox; creating

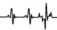

new methods entails destroying the old ones. This loss creates anxiety and can be perceived as a threat to team stability[26]. I suspect that physicians are particularly sensitive to this paradox, and this sensitivity is likely to explain the reluctance of many health care providers to embrace change[1]. In my experience, nurses are more open to change, and nurses who have close working relationships with physicians should be encouraged to coax their physician teammates to at least give change a try. Coaches can also encourage team members to overcome this natural anxiety and embrace approaches that have the potential to improve performance. Teams also may focus on relatively trivial issues to avoid confronting major operational changes. An outside coach can identify these avoidance behaviors and encourage the team to adopt necessary improvements.

3. *Knowledge and skill*—a potential problem in many teams is excessive input from team members whose skill and knowledge may be inappropriately overestimated based on seniority, gender, ethnicity, and/or personality. Team members are subconsciously susceptible to social stereotypes. For example, both men and women perceive that women are less capable in mathematics. Sadly, such stereotypes can create a self-fulfilling prophecy, because if a woman believes she cannot be good in math she may avoid the subject[26]. Similarly, nurses—no matter what their educational accomplishments—often hesitate to actively contribute on teams containing physicians. It is critical that coaches watch for and correct stereotyping. Team members need to be encouraged to base their assessment of skills and knowledge on objective observations.

Because medical team members frequently "pimp" each other (quiz each other on the latest medical facts and management approaches), team members usually quickly assess who possesses the greatest medical knowledge. However, on some medical teams, the loudest and most aggressive personalities may prevail, and their emphatic misstatements may not be immediately discovered. Coaches need to encourage those who are more modest and understated to contribute actively to medical management decisions and procedural plans. The coach should try to ensure that every voice on the team is being heard.

When to Coach

As shown in **Figure 4.7**, coaches need to accomplish different goals at different times in the life of a team. When the team first forms and has not worked together or established routines, the role of the coach should be to reinforce the goals of the team and provide strong motivation. At this juncture the coach should primarily serve as a cheerleader. As the team matures and reaches its midpoint, it often feels the need to make changes and improve its operating procedures and protocols. The midpoint is the ideal time for the coach to serve as a consultant by reviewing strategy and assisting the team in formulating more efficient operating procedures. This is a time to encourage team members to reflect on their performance and brainstorm regarding potential improvements. Another good time to discuss strategy is during periods where there is a lull or downturn in the work requirements of the team. During such periods, the team is more relaxed and can more readily reflect on team performance. These are ideal times to share performance measures and discuss milestones. The team should be asking, "Where are we as a team, and where do we hope to be at the end of our time together?" Finally, at the time the team completes its task, the primary role of the coach is to help the team learn from their successes and their failures. What did the team do well and what could have been improved?

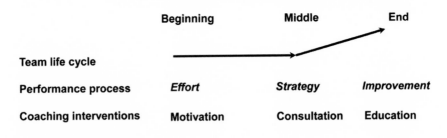

Adapted from Hachman, R. Leading Teams pg. 178

Figure 4.7. Time line for team coaching

How to Coach

A good coach acts as a mirror that reflects back to the team their collective behaviors. Whenever possible, the coach should identify and reward good behaviors. Outstanding coaches create conditions that allow the team to discover their own lessons. They ask open-ended questions that encourage team members to mindfully review how they are conducting their work. What did the team members like about their last meeting, and what did they believe could be improved? Effective coaching focuses on the work itself, not on interpersonal interactions or personalities. If behavior norms are broken, the coach can identify these infractions and then allow the team to enforce these transgressions. Remember that no one personal coaching style is preferred. Coaches should be true to themselves and should not try to emulate another famous coach or personality. Team members quickly recognize unauthentic behavior. Finally, the coach may be tempted to assist the team in identifying resources and removing roadblocks; however, the coach should not be distracted from his/her primary role. The role of the coach is to enhance teamwork, not to help perform the team's work.

> **Case 4.6.** As my first step for improving work rounds, I met with the rounding group. With the group's input, a specific measurable goal was agreed upon: timely (two hours or less) multidisciplinary rounds that ensured active participation by nurses, pharmacists, the case manager, medical students, residents, patients, and patient families. We also agreed upon our primary mission: safe, efficient, patient-centered care of the highest possible quality. The residents agreed to shorten and consistently structure their case presentations. Norms were agreed upon:
>
> 1. Work would be shared, and no resident would leave the hospital until the team's tasks for the day were completed.
> 2. Everyone would be treated with respect and encouraged to participate.
> 3. No one was to break from rounds except in a true emergency.
> 4. Every patient was the team's patient, and core members were responsible to know the key details of every patient on the team.

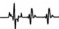

During the second week together, our team was tested. A frightened and ashen-faced twenty-two-year-old woman was admitted after the painless passage of a huge amount of dark red blood from her rectum into the toilet. At an outside hospital she had required eight units of blood (over three-forths of her total blood volume) to maintain her blood pressure. On arrival to our ward, her bleeding had stopped and endoscopy from above and below (gastroscopy and colonoscopy) failed to reveal the source of her bleeding.

Our third-year student reviewed the medical studies on asymptomatic gastrointestinal bleeding and discovered that this form of bleeding was almost always due to a leaking intestinal wall blood vessel. Based on this discussion, we insisted the gastroenterologists and surgeons immediately meet with us to come up with a plan to identify and surgically repair her leaking vessel. We knew she could suddenly begin bleeding again and warned our bedside nurses to have blood ready to administer.

We contacted each of the three gastroenterologists who had previously seen her. Each told us they were no longer responsible for her care. We realized they didn't want to be part of our team! They informed us that a fourth gastroenterologist who had just returned from jury duty was in charge. We insisted that he see this beautiful young woman immediately. Fifteen minutes after his visit, her sheets became stained with bright red blood. She was again actively bleeding. Our team sprung into action. As her blood pressure dropped to seventy, our bedside nurses hung blood and established two intravenous lines to ensure we could provide rapid blood infusion. Our team resident reviewed the care orders, and our student stayed with this frightened young woman and her mother to comfort them. The gastroenterologist contacted a highly experienced surgeon. Our intern, student, and nurses quickly wheeled our patient to the OR, where both our intern and student attended her surgery. The bleeding vessel was identified, and a three-inch section of her bowel containing the leaking vessel was resected. After the total loss of twelve units of blood, our young woman was cured. We knew our fast actions had saved her life.

Case 4.6 represents a continuation of **Case 4.1**. As the conclusion of this case illustrates, effective teamwork can save lives. I should point out that some of the details of this case have been altered to protect confidentiality; however, the description of how our teammates worked together accurately reflected our actions.

We identified our patient's problem as a team and together decided on the most effective course of action. I, as the senior physician and coach, assigned our medical student to search the medical literature and facilitated our team's discussion of her illness. Because everyone on our team clearly understood this young woman's disease and the proper approach to her problem, we were able to recruit a gastroenterologist to temporarily join our team, and he contacted an expert surgeon to identify and surgically correct her leaking blood vessel.

Because our work rounds had included the bedside nurses, they were prepared for emergency blood loss and performed admirably. Our intern immediately took responsibility for escorting our bleeding patient to the operating room and observed the surgery to ensure the surgeon had all the information available to assist her in locating the leaking vessel. No one person could have accomplished all of these tasks. It took a carefully organized and trained health care team.

As our patient left the hospital, we presented her a card congratulating her for surviving her life-threatening illness and gave her a small medal as a memento to wear around her neck. She will always be part of our team, and we will never forget her bravery and miraculous recovery.

Key Points about Coaching

- Coaches should focus primarily on operational issues, not interpersonal issues.
  - Effort—identify social loafers, who
    - are a major cause of process loss;
    - distract the team from its primary goals; and
    - diminish team spirit.
  - Performance strategy—identify avoidance of new strategies.
    - Be aware of the innovation paradox:

- Fear of the new, which requires destroying the old

- Perceived as a threat to team stability
  - Knowledge and skill—teams may fail to utilize the skills and knowledge within the team.
    - Encourage objective assessment of team member skills.
    - Identify and correct social stereotyping.

- Coaches have different goals at different times in the team's lifespan.
  - Beginning—motivation
  - Middle—strategy review and corrections
  - End—education and performance review
    - Ask what went well.
    - Ask what could be improved.

- Good coaches act as mirrors, ask open-ended questions, and are true to their authentic characters.

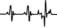

Teamwork and Sharing the Ball
Can Lead to True Joy at Work

Case 4.7. The University of Florida basketball team is playing in the men's 2007 NCAA Championship game against Ohio State. Smiling, the six-foot-eleven center, Joakim Noah, inbounds the ball to shooting guard Lee Humphrey, who quickly passes to point guard, Taurean Green. Green appears determined, yet seems to be close to laughing as he dribbles toward the offensive basket and then passes to six-foot-ten forward, Al Horford. Horford immediately passes to the other forward, six-foot-nine Corey Brewer. With an infectious broad grin, Brewer passes back to Green, slices through the defenders and bounds high above the rim as Green, with pinpoint accuracy, lofts the ball to him. With uncanny speed, Brewer slams the ball through the net. "Corey Brewer for twoooo!" yells the announcer. The five UF players huddle and congratulate Brewer. Every player has a smile on his

face. What is with these guys? Is this championship game some kind of joke to them? The loyal UF fans know better. The team is in the zone, and they are loving every minute of this game. All five players shared the ball before the score, exemplifying the team's unselfish play. By the conclusion of the game, they had easily defeated Ohio State 84-75.

The UF basketball team won back-to-back NCAA Championships. They outscored their opponents in the tournament by an average of fourteen points. They won eighteen consecutive postseason games, a record only exceeded by John Wooden's UCLA teams from the 1970s. Just like Wooden's famous UCLA teams, these players shared the wealth. All five starters averaged over ten points per game, and at the end of the season finished with point averages that were within 3.3 points of each other. All five players took an equal number of opportunities shooting the ball, Corey Brewer taking the most shots at 9.6 per game, and Joakim Noah taking the fewest at 7.2 per game—a difference of only 2.4 shots per game. This impressive team had played together for

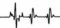

three straight years. Off the court, four of the five—Noah, Brewer, Horford, and Green—were college roommates. As friends and teammates, they enjoyed each other's company and established remarkable team chemistry.

Those of us in health care can take away several important lessons from this championship basketball team. We all need to share responsibility and share the workload. Physicians in particular have a tendency to hog the ball, and such behavior results in poor team performance. Second, members of the health care team should enjoy each other's company. Social interactions outside of work should be encouraged to strengthen team chemistry. When team members like and respect each other, job satisfaction improves, and just like this championship team experienced true joy on the basketball court, the health care team can experience true joy in their work. As exemplified in **Case 4.6**, by sharing the workload, our health care team achieved a championship performance that saved our patient's life, and the two weeks I worked with this team proved to be the most enjoyable two weeks of my medical career.

Key Points about How Effective Teamwork Can Improve Care and Bring Joy to Work

- Sharing the workload and decision making among all the team members increases the likelihood of victory. Don't be a ball hog.

- Enjoy the company of fellow teammates both inside and outside the workplace.

- Experience the joy of true teamwork.

Self-Managing Teams

Experienced teams that have received extensive coaching eventually may be able to manage themselves. If coaches teach team members how to coach, as well as the fundamental supporting elements for teams, then the team can become self-managing. Self-managing teams debrief at the end of every session and review the positives of their performance, as well as the conditions that require change, allowing them to continually improve on their own. This is the ideal team, and in my view the self-managing patient care team is the Holy Grail for medicine. As physicians, nurses, and other care providers become increasing knowledgeable regarding the intricacies of team function, our patient care teams promise to become more and more efficient and promise to provide higher and higher quality care that becomes safer and safer.

Key Points about Self-Managing Teams
- Experienced teams can be taught to coach themselves.
- They debrief daily, asking what went well and what could be improved.
- They are able to continually improve on their own.
- Self-managing teams are the ultimate goal for highly functional patient care teams.

Conclusions

The complexity of modern medical care necessitates that teams rather than lone practitioners provide the care for our patients. Unfortunately, many health care providers are not well schooled in leading and working within teams. This knowledge has now become as necessary as learning how to take a blood pressure measurement and to listen to the heart. In order to benefit from the exciting improvements in coordination, quality, and safety that teams can provide our patients, we must be familiar with the basic requirements for successful teams. Psychologists and business experts have been studying teams for over a decade and now have a rich understanding of team function.

The time has come for all of us in health care to establish the five key conditions known to increase the likelihood of creating productive and highly functional teams (see **Figure 4.1**). We need to

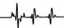

1. provide compelling goals that are significant and relate closely to our overall mission;

2. provide sufficient structure to allow our teams to develop and continually improve;

3. create teams that are bounded and remain together for prolonged periods;

4. provide our teams with appropriate rewards, information, education, and administrative backup to ensure that they prosper; and

5. provide expert coaching that guides each team through continuous cycles of improvement.

Given sufficient time, under these conditions many health care provider teams can become self-managing and self-improving. And these super teams have the potential to lift our entire health care system to new heights in quality, safety, and patient-centered care.

References

1. R. Wageman, D.A. Nunes, J.A. Burruss, and J.R. Hackman. 2008. *Senior Leadership Teams*. Boston, MA: Harvard Business School Press.

2. Institute of Medicine (U.S.). Committee on Quality of Health Care in America. 2001. *Crossing the quality chasm : a new health system for the 21st century*. Washington, D.C.: National Academy Press.

3. M. Hertl, M. Malago, G. Testa, and C. E. Broelsch. 2002. Structural requirements and interactions of transplant centers. *World J Surg* 26 (2):177-180.

4. Linda T. Kohn, Janet Corrigan, Molla S. Donaldson, and Institute of Medicine (U.S.). Committee on Quality of Health Care in America. 2000. *To err is human : building a safer health system*. Washington, D.C.: National Academy Press.

5. M. M. Kim, A. E. Barnato, D. C. Angus, L. F. Fleisher, and J. M. Kahn.

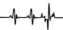
2010. The effect of multidisciplinary care teams on intensive care unit mortality. *Arch Intern Med* 170 (4):369-376.

6. G. Ellrodt, R. Glasener, B. Cadorette, K. Kradel, C. Bercury, A. Ferrarin, D. Jewell, C. Frechette, P. Seckler, J. Reed, A. Langou, and N. Surapaneni. 2007. Multidisciplinary rounds (MDR): an implementation system for sustained improvement in the American Heart Association's Get With The Guidelines program. *Crit Pathw Cardiol* 6 (3):106-116.

7. J. Freeman. 1984. The Tyranny of Structurelessness. In *Untying the Knot - Feminism, Anarchism & Organization*. London, GB: Algate Press.

8. Ruth Rosen. 2000. *The world split open : how the modern women's movement changed America*. New York: Viking.

9. J.R. Hackman. 2002. *Leading Teams*. Boston, MA: Harvard Business Press.

10. I.D. Steiner. 1972. *Group process and productivity*. New York, N.Y.: Academic Press.

11. A. Frankel, M. Leonard, T. Simmonds, C. Haraden, and K.B. Vega. 2009. *The Essential Guide for Patient Safety Officers*. Oakbrook Terrace, IL: Joint Commission Resources, Inc.

12. Joint Commission. 2010. *Sentinel Event Alert #40* 2008 [cited September 12, 2010]. Available from http://www.jointcommission.org/SentinelEvents/ SentinelEventAlert/sea_40.htm.

13. Institute for Safe Medication Practices. 2010. *Survey on workplace intimidation* 2003 [cited September 12, 2010]. Available from https:// ismp.org/Survey/surveyresults/Survey0311.asp.

14. Wihi. 2010. *Unprofessional Behavior Not Permitted Here*: Apple iTunes. Podcast.

15. National Safety Board. 1994.

16. H.C. Foushee, J.K. Lauber, M.M. Baetge, and D.B. Acomb. 1986. Crew factors in flight operations: III. The operation significance of exposure to short-haul air transport operations. In *Technical Memorandum*, No. 88342, edited by Ca Moffet Field, Nasa Ames Research Center.

17. R.M. Wachter. 2008. *Understanding Patient Safety*, Lange Series. New York, NY: McGraw-Hill.

18. L.K. Michaelson, M. Sweet, and D.X. Parmelee. 2008. *Team-based Learning: Small Group Learning's Next Big Step*. Edited by M.D. Svinicki. Vol. 116, *New Directions for Teaching and Learning*. San Francisco, CA: Jossey-Bass.

19. Aacn, Aacom, Aacp, Adea, Aamc, and Asph. 2011. Core Competencies for Interprofessional Collaborative Practice: Report of an Expert Panel.

20. R.C. Ginnett. 1990. Airline cockpit crews. In *Groups That Work (and Those That Don't)*, edited by J.R. Hackman. San Francisco, CA: Jossey-Bass.

21. ———. 1993. Crews as groups: Their formation and leadership. In *Cockpit Resource Management*, edited by E.L. Weiner, B.G. Kanki and J.R. Hackman. Orlando, FL: Academic Press.

22. K. Kanaga, and S Prestridge. 2002. How to Launch a Team. Greensboro, NC: Center for Creative Leadership.

23. D. Leonard. 1999. Chapter 2: Creative Abrasion. In *When Sparks Fly: Igniting Creativity in Groups*, edited by D. Leonard. Boston, MA: Harvard Buisness School Publishing.

24. K.K. Smith, and D.N. Berg. 1987. A Paradoxical Conception of Group Dynamics. *Human Relations* 40:633-657.

25. B. Letourneau. 2004. Managing physician resistance to change. *J Healthc Manag* 49 (5):286-288.

26. S. Begley. 2000. The stereotype trap. *Newsweek*, 66-68.

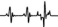
Chapter 4 Exercises

1. Have you worked on a team? Describe the functioning of the team, applying the lessons you have learned in this chapter.

    a. Did your team have all five key supporting conditions?

    b. How well did it function?

    c. What impediments did you encounter?

    d. How would you rate your teammates, and did they have the interpersonal skills to make good team players?

2. Is there a problem or a complex process that you believe would best be managed by forming a team? Why or why not?

3. Describe your vision of the ideal health care team.

    a. What would be your goals and mission?

    b. Who would you pick for your team and why?

    c. Create job descriptions for each member of the team and rate each job for internal motivation assessing: task identity and significance, skill variety, autonomy, and feedback.

    d. What norms do you think would be most important for your team and why?

    e. What will you do about social loafers?

    f. How would you lead the team, and how would you make decisions?

    g. What supporting resources would you ask for and why?

    h. Who would you want to be your coach and why?

$-5-$

WE ALL CAN AND SHOULD LEAD

How Could Effective Leadership Have Improved Mary's Care?

Guiding Questions

1. How much influence can a single leader have on organizational performance?

2. Who can become a health care leader?

3. What personal characteristics should we encourage in health care leaders?

4. What skills are required to become an effective administrator, and why are these skills important for leadership?

5. What is an adaptive leader, and why do we need adaptive health care leaders?

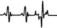

Lost Opportunities

A highly experienced internist was in charge of Mary's care during the initial stages of her hospitalization. Unfortunately for us, he was poorly schooled in leading his rounding team. Based on Mary's poor management, it is likely he never established high expectations for those working with him. His inaction suggests that he never took charge of her care and left decisions to his senior resident or to the consultants. There appeared to be no captain of the ship.

When I visited his office, I quickly realized he was multitasking and that he had failed to establish appropriate priorities. As a consequence, he focused on administrative and research matters and, despite Mary's progressive deterioration, left only a small fraction of his workday to the management of his patients on the ward. In fact, he only visited us briefly once per day during morning rounds. Despite Mary's many complications, he never took time out of his busy afternoons to check on her progress. He never had time to speak to the bedside nurses, who could have shared important insights. As he admitted to me, he had delegated Mary's care to his trainees.

What would have happened if our bedside nurses had seen themselves as leaders and taken charge of what they knew were dysfunctional behaviors on the part of the physicians caring for Mary? What would have happened if they had brought their concerns to the nursing supervisor, who in turn could have contacted the senior physician or his supervisor, the chairman of medicine? If they had called attention to his distracted care, I predict the senior physician would have reprioritized his work schedule. Under these new circumstances, would Mary's blood thinner have been underdosed, would the input of the consultants have been so poorly coordinated, and would treatment with steroids have been delayed? I like to think that the outcome could have been very different. My experience has made me realize that effective nursing as well as physician leadership can spell the difference between life and death.

The Tenuous Nature of Medical Leadership at the Top

In previous decades there was great emphasis on the heroic leader whose charisma, vision, drive, and organizational skills could single-handedly turn around a failing company or a failing organization. However, those who study modern leadership now realize that no single leader has the influence many would like to think he or she possesses[1].

In fact, there is some debate whether a single leader has any control over the fate of an organization. Some suggest that the leader of a large organization is analogous to a driver of a car skidding on ice. As the car careens across the road, guardrails, curbs, lady luck, and God rather than the driver will determine the fate of the car and its passengers[2]. And there is no doubt that external factors powerfully influence an organization's behavior regardless of who is "leading."

Nursing leaders must be sure to create guardrails by building a culture that fosters transparency, open communication, and trust. Methods to improve the culture of health care organizations will be described in the next chapter. Secondly, those passengers traveling with the leader should represent a high-functioning team created by the leader using the methods described in the previous chapter. Effective teams can quickly and expertly advise a leader as to the proper direction to steer.

Those who understand modern leadership now realize that the person at the very top of the. leadership pyramid depends on the leadership of everyone else in the organization. None of us can sit back and assume the head of our health care organization will cure the ills of our care system. We all need to become active participants in bringing about these improvements. Sitting back and complaining simply creates a negative atmosphere and a sense of doom and gloom. We all need to become leaders, and in our leadership roles each of us can make a difference.

Who Should Lead?

Having experienced firsthand the consequences of deficient leadership at the beginning of Mary's hospitalization, as well as outstanding leadership during her recovery in the intensive care unit, I propose a simple definition for leadership: *A health care leader is any person who is able to influence others to objectively improve human health.* This definition empowers janitors as well as administrators, nurses as well as physicians, patients as well as caregivers, and voters as well as politicians to serve as health care leaders.

Returning to Mary's case, what if the neurologist's appointment secretary had taken on a leadership role when I called her for a second appointment? As a leader, she would have attempted to influence the neurologist by telling him that I had requested a new appointment because I felt Mary's condition was worsening. By expressing her concern, she could have influenced the neurologist to see Mary a second time. However, the leadership structure at that time was hierarchical, and everyone was encouraged to "do as they were told." Under these conditions, it is unlikely that her request would have been acted upon. In fact, she probably would have been fired for insubordination. What could have happened if the power structure had been more horizontal and the physician had responded, "If you are concerned, that raises a red flag. Thank you for alerting me to this potential problem, and please make an appointment for Mary later today."

What would have happened if the bedside nurse caring for Mary had acted as a leader and notified the medical attending physician that Mary's anticoagulation levels were low? This very experienced clinician could have checked the laboratory data, increased the blood thinner (heparin) dose, and prevented Mary from developing blood clots in her lungs. However, the nurse was fearful of jeopardizing her working relationship with the medical residents and told us about the subtherapeutic anticoagulation levels only after Mary suffered her complication. These events occurred twenty years ago, and nursing educators and safety experts are now encouraging nurses to speak out when they have a concern.

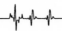

As Mary's husband and a fellow physician faculty member, I also attempted to influence others to improve Mary's care. I spoke with many of the consultants and encouraged them to collaborate. I encouraged the first attending physician to pay greater attention to Mary's case. Unfortunately my actions increased the anxiety of the caregivers and failed to improve her care. I was dismissed as a worried husband, and my concerns were ignored until Mary was transferred to the intensive care unit. Leadership depends on context, and when the culture only encourages top-down leadership, nurses, patients, patient families, ward clerks, and other caregivers lower on the hierarchy are disempowered from influencing others to improve health. They are not allowed to lead.

Key Points about Who Should Lead

- A health care leader is any person who is able to influence others to objectively improve human health.

- Anyone can choose to be a health care leader, including nurses, patients, patient families, ward clerks, and hospital janitors.

- Developing leadership requires the creation of a more horizontal power structure that encourages everyone to lead.

Can I Become a Leader?

Thousands of books have been written on leadership (68,000 titles are listed on Amazon.com), and the underlying premises of leadership are continually changing and evolving[1-4]. A major problem with much of the leadership literature is the absence of a rigorous evidence-based underpinning. Journalists, business consultants, and successful leaders have written experience-based and interview-based books that are often anecdotal and at times self-serving. Nonetheless, these books do contain kernels of wisdom and provide many potentially helpful suggestions.

Two of the most important and exciting realizations are that leadership can be taught and that there is no specific personality type required to be a successful leader. Each person who aspires to become a leader or who is recruited to a leadership position should avoid the temptation to simply emulate an admired leader[5]. This strategy carries the risk of being viewed as disingenuous. Leaders must recognize and use their unique strengths to inspire and lead others. Every leader must remember Shakespeare's adage, "This above all: to thine own self be true"[6]. Some highly successful leaders are quiet, calm, and deliberate in their actions[7], while others are vocal, excitable, and quick to act[8]. As discussed at the very beginning of the chapter, the culture of the organization often plays a far greater role than personality in determining a leader's success.

Key Points about Becoming a Leader
- Leaders are not born; leadership can be taught.

- Any personality type can become a proficient leader.

- Leaders need to be genuine and use their strengths as leaders.
  - Do not simply emulate other leaders.
  - Be true to yourself.

Interpersonal Skills

Case 5.1. Maureen Bisognano, the CEO of the Institute for Health Care Improvement (IHI), is the oldest of nine children from a tightly knit Irish family. Her mother was a nurse, and she followed her mother's example, first serving as an ICU nurse. Her passion for innovation and her love of people led to a meteoric rise up the nursing administrative ladder and subsequently to IHI. While she was in nursing school, her brother developed Hodgkin's disease, and she devoted considerable time caring for him before he died at age twenty-one. Two years later, her deeply admired father died of colon cancer at age fifty-three. These losses brought the family even closer together, and they have shared their sadness and overcome these challenges as a team. Maureen noted that in addition to the tears, there was "lots of fun, lots of laughing, and lots of conversation."

As Maureen steps into a room to present her wisdom, a warmness and genuine interest in her audience is immediately apparent. As she asks questions of the audience, she looks into each person's eyes. Her stories of personal loss and triumph enrapture, and her narrative transfixes the audience. She demonstrates empathy and openness. Her interpersonal skills by anyone's estimation are off the charts. She exemplifies the culture and values of IHI: a focus on joy in work and the continuous engagement of like-minded, like-valued people dedicated to improving health care. All interactions at IHI are transparent. The walls of the offices are glass, and an average of six to seven people work at long counters in each office. No one has his or her own space. Teamwork and "boundarylessness" create "one global brain."[1]

If only we could all be like Maureen Bisognano, the world of health care would be a wonderful environment in which to work. When Maureen greets you, you immediately sense her genuine interest in you as a person. There is immediate eye-to-eye contact, and she always mentions your first name: "Fred, so glad you could be with us today." She can provide even Dale Carnegie a few lessons on social interaction[9]. As exemplified by Maureen, IHI selects employees who display openness, humility, and a willingness to work in teams. Unfortunately, these traits have not always been primary selection criteria for nursing or medical students. Nonetheless, these behaviors can be taught, encouraged, and emulated by student instructors.

Another important interpersonal skill is self-awareness. Each of us needs to take time out and critically evaluate our own behavior. How did I interact with others at the meeting? Did I empower others to speak, or did I dominate the conversation? Too often leaders feel they need to share their expertise and showcase their intellectual powers, and I have been guilty of this behavior. Those in charge need to step back and view themselves as facilitators who encourage others to share their ideas. After all, we know what we think, and as leaders we need to incorporate the ideas of others before making decisions and creating action plans. The most important four words an administrator

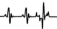

can repeatedly utter are, "What is your opinion?"[10] As Maureen has noted, "I look at how often leaders ask questions versus how often they give answers. Leadership is learning. It's being open to the gifts of the people who work in your organization"[1]. Good leaders empower others.

Key Points about Interpersonal Skills

- Openness (transparency), humility, and a willingness to work with others are critical attributes of the ideal leader.

- Leaders show genuine interest in others.

- To be a good leader, you should be self-aware and review how you interacted with others daily.

- Leaders empower others and primarily listen.

Case 5.2. The chronic illness of his father profoundly affected Thomas's childhood. His father suffered with malignant hypertension, first diagnosed at age thirty-five years. Physicians were helpless when it came to controlling his father's BP of 300/230, and he developed congestive heart failure that impaired his ability to work and walk. His father became extremely depressed, and as a teenager Thomas was required to be his father's caregiver. With tears in his eyes, Thomas recalls how his father suddenly lost consciousness and fell into his arms while they sat together in the living room. His father had suffered a fatal stroke. As Switzerland's secretary of health, Dr. Thomas Zeltner has never forgotten his father's chronic debilitating disease or its disruption of his childhood and family life. This firsthand understanding of chronic illness explains his passion for improving public health. As the secretary of health, he strongly opposed the unseemly lobbying of the cigarette companies to stop the World Health Organization from publicizing the health risks of cigarette smoking. These activities placed Dr. Zeltner number two on the cigarette companies' enemies list. Whenever possible, these powerful companies framed his activities in a negative light, and they continually lobbied for his dismissal. Dr. Zeltner also elicited the enmity of fellow Swiss physicians when he proposed to lower the reimbursement rates for laboratory tests. Fees for blood tests had not changed in over a decade despite dramatic improvements in automation that had reduced expenses. Physicians were outraged and convinced their patients to oppose his new policy. He met with the medical societies to explain his rationale, and at one meeting the audience pummeled him with tomatoes. Their treatment was demeaning, and at times he felt as if the whole country was against him. However, in his heart Thomas Zeltner knew his actions were just and fair, and he stuck by his principles.

Moral Leadership

As Thomas Zeltner's case vividly exemplifies, challenging the status quo takes courage. Despite intense opposition to many of his policies, Thomas proved to be the longest serving secretary of health in Switzerland's history; he served for nineteen years. He nurtured and modified the Swiss health system, making it a model system for the industrialized world. His childhood experiences provided him with the moral backbone to stand up to special interests and to always protect the needs of people like his father. He never lost his strong moral compass[8].

Leaders are symbols of moral unity and should express the values that hold society together. One of a leader's most important goals should be to lift people out of their petty preoccupations and unite them behind strong moral principles[4]. Nursing leaders need to remember Thomas Zeltner's inspirational example and employ objective facts and moral values to guide their actions and to counter the demagoguery and misinformation offered by those who have a major stake in the status quo. We should never lose sight of our ultimate goal: to improve the health of all people. Despite the potential danger of being pummeled by tomatoes, we should try to maintain the highest ethical standards[11] and always do what is right for our patients.

Just like Thomas Zeltner, Michelle Lewis (**Case 5.3**) exhibited remarkable courage in standing up to a physician who had ignored the financial consequences of his actions to his patients. She possessed the strength and self-confidence to repeatedly challenge someone who was higher in the power structure. High-functioning organizations accept such challenges when they further the primary goals of the institution, and the physician's supervisor as well as Michelle's supervisor backed her. Nurses will frequently be called upon to defend the interests of their patients, and they should remember Michelle's and Thomas's examples. Be courageous when your patients' welfare is at stake.

Key Points about Ethical (Moral) Leadership

- Leaders are symbols of moral unity.

- A strong moral compass is critical for health care leaders.

- No matter what the personal cost, we should all try to maintain the highest ethical standards.

- We should never lose sight of our ultimate goal: to improve the health of all people.

- We need to be courageous.

Case 5.3. Michelle Lewis had always wanted to be a nurse. Her mother quit nursing school and always regretted not entering the profession. She encouraged her daughter at an early age to become a nurse. As a young woman, Michelle rebelled against her mother's wishes. However, her desire to become a nurse was never extinguished, and at age thirty-seven, after raising three daughters, she entered nursing school and proved to be an exceptional student. Upon graduating, she became an inpatient oncology nurse; however, after ten years she realized she desired a job that allowed her to spend more time teaching patients and following their full hospital course. She became an oncology case manager and spent hours helping patients manage their insurance, instructing them how to apply for Medicaid, assisting them with

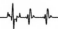

their bills and medication prescriptions, finding them housing, and placing them in appropriate long-term care facilities.

In her role, she noticed that one physician was ignoring the insurance rules for hospital admission and admitting patients without appropriate medical justification. The consequence was that the insurance companies refused to pay, and these patients were forced to personally pay their bills. The financial drain on patients was devastating, but when Michelle informed the physician, he ignored her pleas and continued his unapproved admissions. Michelle notified the physician's supervisor, and initially the physician changed his practice. However, within weeks he returned to his old practices, causing financial harm to his patients. Michelle again intervened; he again changed his behavior but again relapsed. Michelle did not give up, and eventually the physician permanently gave up his old admitting practices but complained bitterly to colleagues about her actions. Michelle knew in her heart that she was doing what was best for her patients.

How Do I Become an Effective Leader?

Leadership should be evaluated based on objective measures, not simply on process, personality, or popularity. The effective leader not only creates strategies but also orchestrates action. Effective leaders must be effective managers, and according to Peter Drucker—a renowned and highly regarded business consultant—there are four elements required for effective management[12]. Based on my personal experiences, I have added a fifth element that I believe is critical for health care.

1. Time Management

Results are the currency of superior leadership, and to achieve results, effective leaders allot sufficient time. As John Wooden, the most successful college basketball coach of past century, often stated during his carefully scheduled basketball practices, "What can you never get back? Time."[13] Good leaders closely monitor their time and reduce the time wasted on unimportant projects. To have a significant impact on people, effective leaders block off sufficient time (one to one and a half hours minimum) to engage and interact with them[12]. Similar consolidations of free time are required to attain a full understanding of a problem and to create successful solutions. Often excessive time is spent interacting with others rather than accomplishing the expected goals. We all need to be more like "Lord Heart of the Matter," Harry Hopkins, head of the Work Projects Administration (WPA), major architect of the New Deal, and valued advisor to Franklin D. Roosevelt. At the end of his career, he suffered from terminal stomach cancer. Despite only having sufficient energy to work a few hours a day, he continued to play an integral role in guiding the United States during WWII[12].

Another important strategy for effectively managing time is to establish priorities. Most human beings can efficiently perform only one task at a time. Individuals who attempt to multitask—that is, go from task to task, working on each project for a brief period, and trying to advance multiple projects simultaneously—often fail to accomplish their goals despite expending extra effort. Efficiency experts recommend completing one project before moving to another. The effective leader decides which project is most important to accomplish first; in other words, he or she does "first things first."

The senior physician who first cared for Mary in the hospital did not manage his time well and did not establish priorities. He attempted to juggle departmental administrative tasks, research projects, and Mary's care. As a consequence, he was unable to devote his full attention to Mary's illness. Effective nurse leaders and bedside nurses carefully schedule their time and devote sufficient time to the activities that really matter, the activities that further their ultimate goal, which is to provide the best possible care for each patient. As recommended by Toyota Production System managers, we all need to ask ourselves, "Will this activity be of benefit to our patients?" If the answer is no, this activity should be minimized or eliminated.

2. Make a Unique Contribution

No matter how modest a person's stature in an organization, all effective leaders focus on what they can contribute. We each need to ask ourselves, "What can I and no one else do, that if done really well will make a difference to my organization?"[12] In deciding on their unique contribution, effective leaders ask themselves, "What is my passion? What is important to me?" This requires looking into one's soul and asking, "What do I value?"[8] When it comes to health care, the meaningfulness of our work is ever apparent: improving the health of others. This goal is internally rewarding, and caring for others brings true meaning to each caregiver's life. To be effective, each nurse leader must understand his or her unique contribution and ensure that his or her contribution is usable. To accomplish this task, each of us must understand the needs, the limitations, and perceptions of others and be assured they understand our contribution.

For example, in Mary's case our bedside nurses were always approachable and empathetic. We found several of the nurses to be very personable, cheerful, and positive in their approaches. They never gave up hope, and they allowed me to lean on their emotional shoulders during the period when I truly believed Mary's life was over. They had what is sometimes termed an outstanding bedside manner. I remain grateful that they were able to share with us their unique interpersonal skills.

3. Focus on Strengths

Case 5.4. Being the twelfth of sixteen children in her family, African American, and a resident of the small rural town of Reddick, Florida, Rose Rivers had "not expected much" of her life. Being from such a large family with limited resources, she quickly learned to be independent and resourceful. At age sixteen she sought employment in a local nursing home, hoping to become a dietary clerk; however the director told her they needed a nurse's aide, and she accepted the position.

Impressed with her patient skills, the director encouraged her to return to school to earn a nursing degree. Her best friend discouraged Rose from applying, telling her, "You're wasting your time." She didn't listen. Rose applied and was accepted. From there she never looked back. From an RN in a local hospital in Ocala, Florida, she moved to the Shands Hospital, where she earned her bachelor's, master's, and PhD degrees at the University of Florida.

While at Shands, the vice president for nursing and patient services, Sue Ellen Pinkerton, took Rose under her wing and assigned her ever more challenging administrative roles. Rose was chosen as a Robert Wood Johnson Executive Nurse Fellow, and this experience opened her eyes. "I didn't realize that I was so bound by traditional ways of doing things and so bound by solid lines of authority. I came to realize that I was the one that I was waiting for."

When Sue Ellen Pinkerton expanded her scope, Rose was appointed vice president of nursing, and she immediately reached for the sky. When making appointment decisions, she always advanced those with the "greatest strengths." She followed her personal definition of success: "be good to do good." She established an effective nursing leadership course that allowed her nurse leaders to become experts, and they "completed the course knowing that they can."

Despite trepidation and doubts by those close to her, she chose to seek Magnet status for their nursing service. This is the most prestigious designation, and by focusing and building on each nurse's personal strengths in 2003, Rose and her inspired nursing team achieved this coveted designation.

As emphasized by **Case 5.4**, all effective leaders focus on and build on the strengths of others. They avoid devoting significant time to minimizing weaknesses and instead focus on maximizing strengths. They staff for strength rather than staffing to avoid weakness because the end result of the second

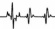

strategy will be mediocrity. As Rose Rivers emphasized, leaders should always pick those with the "greatest strengths," and by building on these strengths, you too can guide your organization to reach the equivalent of Magnet status.

One of the starkest examples of mistakenly choosing to minimize weakness occurred during the America's Civil War. For the first three years of the war, Abraham Lincoln chose generals who had no major weaknesses. The consequence was repeated defeats by the Confederacy despite the Union's clear superiority in men and equipment. Robert E. Lee, the head of the Confederate army, had staffed for strength, and when making his selections, he had ignored his generals' weaknesses. He always recognized and built on his generals' strengths. Only after Lincoln staffed for strength and hired a general not afraid to go on the offensive, Ulysses Grant, did the Union's fortunes in war take a turn for the better[12].

Remember that strong people can also have strong weaknesses. (General Grant was a known heavy drinker). They have both high peaks and low valleys, and no one can be strong in all areas. The leader who worries about what a man or women cannot do rather than about what he or she can do is a weak leader. I did not witness how Mary's senior physician and team resident supervised her intern; however, based on his poor performance, I suspect they focused on his weaknesses rather than bringing out his strengths.

4. Make Effective Decisions

Most students of leadership agree that the most important leadership skill is the ability to make effective decisions. The first step is to gather all the pertinent information and to solicit opinions from all involved parties. Most people do not start out with facts but rather with opinions, and when asked to research the facts, too often they seek only the facts that support their opinions. This approach is particularly problematic in medicine, and physicians—and I suspect nurses too—often utilize personal opinion rather than utilizing the wealth of medical information available to them. And patients too often do not properly research the alternative approaches to their illness or obtain a second opinion. They simply abdicate decisions to their physician. Similarly nurses often blindly follow the physician's orders without respectfully questioning the reasoning behind the physician's decisions. Nurses can and should contribute to the therapeutic and diagnostic plans for their patients and inquire about the medical evidence supporting each decision. When it comes to health care decisions, objective evidence should prevail whenever possible and objective methods are available for assessing the quality of medical studies and the strength of specific recommendations.

Another important aspect of decision making is the ability to differentiate a straightforward or generic problem from an unusual or unique problem. In the case of a patient's complaint, does the patient have a straightforward problem that can be handled using a standard management protocol, or does the complaint represent an unusual problem? In Mary's case, the neurologist assumed that her nerve injury was caused by trauma, a generic problem that he frequently encountered, and he recommended tincture of time to allow the nerve to heal on its own.

In reality, Mary had a very unusual allergic reaction to penicillin that had caused her immune system to attack her nerves, and treatment with corticosteroids would have prevented further injury. Similarly, the internists who first treated Mary assumed she had the generic problem of thrombophlebitis (blood clots in her legs) and simply treated her with blood thinner. They ignored the high level of eosinophils in her peripheral blood, as well as her skin lesions, which strongly suggested a severe allergic reaction.

Similarly nurses and nurse practitioners need to be cautious about inadvertently labeling a unique problem as a generic one. As they gain experience and see more and more specific generic complaints they will develop pattern recognition and will sense when a patient does not exactly fit the pattern of the generic disease. When a nurse senses a case is atypical, it will be important for them to seek help from an experienced physician who has expertise related to the atypical complaint.

Once a problem has been clearly defined, the decision must be converted to an action. Without action, a decision only represents a good intention, and too many leaders hesitate to act. Action may take courage, and as discussed above, courage is a very important attribute for nursing and physician leaders who

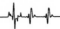
want to bring about constructive change. In Mary's situation, those managing her case failed to act until she was close to death, and there is concern by many health care critics that our administrative leaders will fail to act until our health system has suffered a similar fate[14].

Finally, after taking action, effective leaders obtain feedback that tests the effectiveness of their actions. Without objective performance measurements, meaningful improvement is impossible. Feedback allows the leader to modify his or her decisions when the original action has unintended consequences or fails to achieve the envisioned goals. In Mary's case, all measures of Mary's health progressively worsened; however, the physicians ignored this feedback until she was transferred to the intensive care unit.

As was discussed in Chapter 1, our health care leaders (all of us) have received objective feedback that our system is killing large numbers of patients unnecessarily, is far more expensive than other industrial nations, and ranks thirty-seventh with regards to performance. It is very clear that we all need to change our strategies and act in new ways.

5. Be a Frontline Leader

Case 5.5. B.J. Sullivan has been a nurse for thirty-six years. She began as a floor nurse but then became a nurse recruiter. She enjoyed recruiting new nurses but realized that her real love was directly caring for patients, and she eventually returned to be a bedside nursing. "I am proud to be a bedside nurse. God puts you where he needs you." She clearly loves being with her patients. She remembers fondly one of her favorite patients, a ninety-four-year-old man with 90° kyphosis. She spent thirty minutes positioning pillows to provide proper support. Upon her completion of the task, he warmly thanked her, saying, "This is the first time I have been comfortable in a long time." He described his narrowly escaped death as a child. His parents' friends in London urged the entire family to stay for a longer visit, and as a consequence they missed their voyage on the Titanic. B.J. loves working with the elderly because of their insightful perspective on life. "Not a single

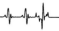

day goes by without me learning something new." When asked what she felt made a good nurse leader, she enthusiastically described the leadership team on her floor. "Whenever I have a problem, one of our nurse unit leaders is there, listening and helping. They work beside us and pitch in." She always feels supported, and in turn she continually advises and helps her fellow nurses. She loves to teach the younger nurses the fine points of effective bedside nursing care.

B.J. Sullivan is a frontline leader. She shares her wisdom and experience with the younger nurses on the floor and leads by example. Her very positive outlook and love for nursing is infectious. Furthermore, she describes her nurse managers in glowing terms because, just like the supervisors at Southwest Air, they remain on the floor, observing and listening and working alongside the bedside nurses when additional help is required. Health care is all about our patients, and to understand the roadblocks and frustrations of bedside and clinic nurses, all administrators should spend time on the floors and in the clinics, observing and listening to the concerns of those working on the front lines.

Key Points about Being an Effective Leader
- Effectively manage your time.
  - Block one to one and a half hours time for each important task.
    - Use blocks of time for
      - policy decisions and
      - mentoring those you are leading.
  - Establish priorities.
    - Don't multitask.
    - Complete one task before going to another.

- Focus on your unique contribution.
  - Ask yourself, "What can I uniquely contribute to advancing the goals of my organization?"
  - Follow your passion. Ask, "What do I value?"
  - Make sure your contribution is usable.

- Focus on your strengths and the strengths of others.
  - Do not hire to avoid weaknesses; it results in mediocrity.
  - Don't worry about what a person cannot do; worry about what they can do well.

- Make effective decisions.
  - Most people start with opinions, but you need to explore all the objective facts.
  - Determine whether you are dealing with a generic or unique problem.
  - Once a decision is made, act.
  - After acting, obtain feedback and change course when necessary.

- Be a frontline manager.

Strategies for Distributive Leadership

When a leader insists on managing every major function of an organization and creating a wheel and spoke model for leadership, there will be no increase in the leadership quotient of the organization. Furthermore, this leadership approach leads to eventual burnout of the person at the center of the wheel (see **Figure 5.1**). Leadership should be encouraged and taught throughout our health centers. The Mayo Clinic has embraced a distributive leadership model that allows all members of the organization to learn leadership skills by doing. One or two individuals rarely make decisions at the Mayo Clinic. Rather, committees are empowered to direct the institution, and at any one time there are eighty committees charged with establishing specific policies and protocols[15].

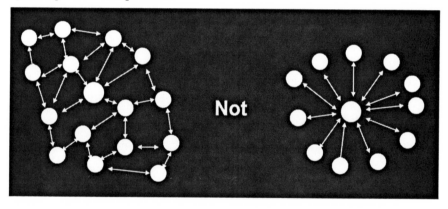

Figure 5.1. Distributive versus centralized leadership. Leadership must be distributed throughout the organization, not centered around a single individual like spokes on a wheel. The right hand model leads to burnout and fails to increase the leadership quotient.

Compared to decisions made by a single leader, the team decision-making process is slower and has been criticized as being inefficient; however, the critics ignore an important added dividend: decision by committee encourages buy-in and shortens the adoption phase. By applying the team skills described in Chapter 4, the efficiency of these teams can be improved and decisions streamlined. The critics of team decision making must keep in mind that when dictums come from on high, frontline employees often resist the proposed changes, and adoption could be delayed for months to years or, even worse, permanently ignored.

To further encourage a distributive leadership, the Mayo Clinic maintains a policy of rotational leadership. Leaders generally remain in one position for five to ten years and then are expected to move to a new administrative role. This policy encourages continual learning and renewal among its leaders and provides the institution with leaders who have a broad overview of the institution. By rotating leaders to new positions, department loyalty and the tendency toward silo formation is minimized. Most importantly, this policy creates opportunities for new leaders to be recruited to positions of authority and allows the Mayo Clinic to build its leadership quotient.

The Mayo Clinic has a strong commitment to its employees and generally promotes from within. The combination of participatory decision making and upward mobility creates internal motivation and high job satisfaction, and as a consequence, the institution-wide employee turnover rate is only 2.5 percent as compared to most medical centers, where the average annual turnover ranges from 9–30 percent[15, 16].

To further invest in the growth of its employees, the Clinic has established a formal career and leadership program that consists of four modules. Module one for newly appointed staff consists of three key areas of instruction: lessons in Mayo Clinic's heritage and values, followed by instruction on personal development and teamwork. Module two is designed for newly appointed leaders and members of leadership teams and includes four areas of instruction: your role as a leader, maximizing financial performance to achieve Mayo's mission, leading organizational change, and developing people. To improve the performance of experienced leaders, module three teaches how to build a culture of quality, safety, and service and simultaneously reduce waste. Finally, for their senior leadership, module four covers strategic planning and objective measurement to assess progress[15]. This program not only ensures a highly skilled leadership pool but also establishes explicit expectations for leaders and a clear path for career advancement.

> **Key Points about Distributive Leadership**
> - Avoid the wheel and spoke model of leadership.
>
> - Encourage the formation of working teams for major decisions:
>   - Slows decision making
>   - Improves adoption because employee buy-in
>   - Increases the organization's leadership quotient
>
> - Rotate leadership positions every in five- to ten-year cycles.
>
> - Create leadership training modules for different stages of leadership.
>
> - Create explicit career paths for leaders.

Picking the Right People for Your Team or Organization

One skill that all leaders acknowledge as being critical for successful organizations is picking the right people to be part of your team. Those who are selected represent the organization's future, and if chosen wisely and trained properly, these new recruits will become the organization's future leaders.

Two of the most important traits that are not always emphasized in choosing nurses and other health care employees are industriousness and enthusiasm[13]. Industriousness connotes more than simply showing up on time and punching the clock. It suggests full engagement and a clear focus on the task at hand. This approach is critical for providing the best patient care, and medical caregivers need to embrace hard work, and when in the hospital, they need to devote 100 percent effort and attention to their patients. Enthusiasm is equally important because without enthusiasm, work is drudgery. Nurses, physicians, and other caregivers must enjoy their work and love what they do. Without enthusiasm, there cannot be true industriousness, and success virtually always requires both of these cornerstones.

As both a trainer of physicians and nurses and as a family member of a patient, I have come to realize that attitude is often more important than aptitude. Too often caregivers allow the frustrations of our dysfunctional systems, personal problems, and negative interactions with others to dampen their enthusiasm. Too often caregivers focus on leaving work early rather than focusing on the joy of the present moment. Patients should expect their caregivers to enthusiastically devote 100 percent effort to their care. And when patients or their family members experience apathy and laziness on the part of their caregivers, they naturally become concerned because, as I experienced firsthand, this behavior often leads to the distracted and error-prone care.

Other important characteristics include loyalty, friendship, and co-operation. Cooperation is particularly important in health care. When a caregiver insists on his or her own way rather than the best way, patient care is compromised. An effective management team must be able to share ideas and together create the ideal treatment plan for each patient. With the exception of emergency situations, autocracy should be discouraged, and cooperation should be emphasized and rewarded.

Friendship is rarely discussed in medicine; however, genuine friendship greatly enhances team spirit and job satisfaction. Loyalty to the team and to the team's patients creates a nurturing atmosphere where trust increases, and it allows the formation of a zone of psychological safety where everyone feels comfortable sharing their ideas. Loyalty should prevent the all-too-common practice of disparaging a teammate or patient behind his or her back. When overworked and frustrated health care providers blame fellow team members rather than the malfunctioning systems, they undermine their teams.

When it comes to nurses and doctors, honesty is a trait that has generally been taken for granted. However, too often nurses and physicians cover up their mistakes and lapses rather than confessing that they made an error. Their desire to always appear competent, rather than accepting the reality that we are all imperfect, encourages half-truths and cover-ups. Nurses as well as physicians and other caregivers should remember to always tell it like it is, not how you wish it to be. Without truthfulness, errors may persist and result

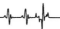

in irreparable patient harm.

Self-control is a critical trait when working in teams. The most effective nurses and physicians remain calm and don't let anxiety and frustration color their judgment. Too often more senior nurses, as well as physicians, fail to control their anger and lash out at those below them when a problem arises. As discussed earlier, the majority of cases delays, oversights, and errors are the consequence of bad systems rather than bad people. Loss of self-control harms a leader's image and distracts others from their focus on patient care. Loss of self-control destroys morale and endangers our patients.

Inquisitiveness is a particularly important trait for modern health care providers. Each of us needs to continually ask why. All caregivers need to know how to generate a hypothesis and test it. These fundamental skills are critical for creating effective diagnostic and treatment plans and for generating permanent solutions to recurrent problems within our health care system, including preventable errors that harm our patients.

Too often nurses step back and allow physicians to ask all the questions. However, because they are the ones who are constantly at the bedside, nurses are the most likely to observe signs or symptoms that may not fit with the proposed diagnosis. They are also the most likely to encounter problems with equipment and procedures that may lead to patient harm. By asking, "Why is my patient having this symptom?" or "Why is this pulse oxymeter intermittently malfunctioning?" nurses can call the management team's attention to unexpected changes in a patient's clinical presentation and alert the appropriate administrator to possible equipment malfunctions.

Having experienced firsthand the emotional support of our bedside nurses as I prepared for Mary's death, I can unequivocally state that empathy and compassion are among the most important personal traits nurses should possess. As the longtime nursing administrator, Rose Rivers (see **Case 5.4**) commented to me, the "ability to interact with humans with heart" is one of the most fundamental traits she looks for when choosing new nursing recruits. "The ability to love, to do right by your patient"[17] is the essence of nursing. Effective caregivers look through the eyes of their patients and visibly show that they care.

> **Key Points about Team Selection in Nursing**
> - Industriousness and enthusiasm help to create joy at work.
>
> - Friendship and loyalty encourage cooperation and eliminate backbiting.
>
> - Honestly telling in like it is, not the way you want to be, is critical for reducing errors.
>
> - Self-control is important for fostering team work.
>
> - Initiative and being inquisitive, always asking why, encourage continual improvements in care.
>
> - Empathy and compassion are the essence of nursing.

What Is an Adaptive Leader, and Why Do We Need Adaptive Leaders in Health Care?

> There is nothing more difficult to carry out, nor more doubtful of success, nor more dangerous to handle, than to initiate a new order of things. For the reformer has enemies all who profit by the old order, and only lukewarm defenders in all those who would profit from the new order. This lukewarmness arises partly from fear of their adversaries who have the law in their favor; and partly from the incredulity of mankind, who do not truly believe in anything new until they have had actual experience of it.
>
> —Niccolo Machiavelli, 1515

As detailed in the preceding chapters, there are many dysfunctional conditions within our modern health care delivery systems. However, based on the seeming lack of urgency among many of our health care leaders, these systems cannot be too dysfunctional, or those working within them would be more eager to bring about change. As Machiavelli points out, change is dangerous, and those in leadership positions often reach their levels of authority because they have avoided changing "the order of things."

If we hope to truly improve how we care for our patients, we will require a new type of leadership known as adaptive leadership. "Adaptive leadership is the practice of mobilizing people to tackle tough problems and thrive."[18] Adaptive leaders take a Darwinian approach to business and societal problems. They preserve the useful operational or structural components and discard the maladaptive ones. Then they rearrange the original components to create systems that allow the organization to flourish or thrive. An adaptive leader is capable of diagnosing specific problems by asking the right questions of those directly confronting the problem and by carefully observing the processes that require change. Once the problem is appropriately diagnosed, the adaptive leader intervenes using strategies that take into account the context, the leader's personal abilities, and the abilities of those required to undergo change (see **Figure 5.2**).

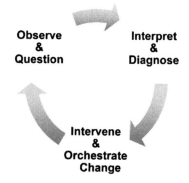

Figure 5.2. The adaptive leadership process (adapted from Heifetz et al.[18])

Adaptive leaders build on the past rather than discarding it. And adaptive reorganization is exciting because change is guided by experimentation and requires multiple iterations that involve the input of multiple stakeholders. Effective adaptive leaders incorporate diverse ideas. They understand that the resulting new adaptations will displace prior processes and positions and should be carried out incrementally. Adaptive change almost always takes time.

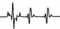

Case 5.6. Kathleen Long, dean of the College of Nursing at the University of Florida for the past sixteen years, knew she wanted to be a nurse by the end of her high school years. Her mother was a very caring and talented nurse, and her father was a dentist. He was the first in his family to earn a college degree, and he repeatedly reminded his children, including his two daughters, that education was the one thing no one could ever take from them. His strong encouragement and that of a forward-thinking high school principal convinced Kathleen to complete her BS in nursing and to continue on for an MS in nursing, followed soon thereafter by a PhD in behavioral science at Johns Hopkins. Upon completing her final degree, ignoring the warnings of her professors at Johns Hopkins that her "professional career might be over" if she accepted a position at the rural Montana State University College of Nursing, she opted for the position, encouraged by then dean, Dr. Anna Shannon, who became a lifelong mentor.

At Montana State, Kathleen was given support for advancement in her faculty roles, as well as administrative opportunities; she became dean in 1990 after the retirement of her mentor and a national search. Over the years, Kathleen had many leadership opportunities at the national level and espoused the lessons of her father to embrace higher education. She led several national initiatives to encourage nursing organizations to move toward requiring a four-year college education and beyond for professional nurses.

She encountered strong emotional resistance, and to this day vividly recalls being challenged by a prominent nursing leader who favored continuing two- year RN degrees. "I don't see why you have to extinguish our little light so that you can shine more brightly." What should Kathleen say? She knew that objective studies were beginning to demonstrate better patient outcomes when the nursing workforce was better educated. Wasn't that the point? Shouldn't we do what is best for our patients? She was stunned and did not respond because she knew objective facts would eventually prevail.

How can nurses provide leadership in the complex environment of today's health care systems without at least four-years of college? Nurses are now expected to seamlessly communicate with highly educated physicians and are being asked to become more involved in every phase of patient care. In her mind and in the minds of many of today's nursing leaders, more education must serve as the foundation for advancing professional nursing and improving patient care.

From her early childhood, Kathleen Long's father emphasized education, and Kathleen has devoted her career to improving nursing education. As a new graduate of her PhD program, she took a risk leaving the hallowed halls of Johns Hopkins to move to a rural nursing school to be with an admired mentor. She successfully advanced in her educational career and was able to encourage a major change within nursing. She, like many nurse educators, has realized that with the increasing complexity of medicine, as well as the new emphasis on a team-based medical care, nurses require a higher level of education. Through her leadership positions in multiple national nursing organizations, Kathleen has championed a four-year bachelor of science degree as the minimum requirement for professional nurses. The consequence would be the discontinuation of two-year degree nursing schools, and she has encountered considerable resistance from those favoring the status quo. Recognizing the changing needs of the nursing profession, Kathleen Long has served as a courageous adaptive leader.

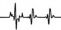

> **Key Points about Adaptive Leadership**
> - "Adaptive leadership is the practice of mobilizing people to tackle tough problems and thrive."
>
> - Adaptive leaders
>   - keep useful operations and systems and discard maladaptive ones;
>   - rearrange old systems to create new, more effective ones;
>   - observe and question;
>   - interpret and diagnose; and
>   - intervene to bring about meaningful change.
>
> - Adaptive change allows organizations to achieve their goals and allows people to thrive.

GATEWAY

ENTER

SEVEN

http://bit.ly/tlhBpx

Differentiating Technical from Adaptive Change

Organizations and systems must undergo two types of change to improve. Technical change requires the application of solutions using current knowledge and can be achieved by applying the appropriate expertise. A consultant can be hired to design technical fixes, and these technical changes can be implemented using the organization's current structures, procedures, and traditional ways of doing things. Adaptive change, on the other hand, is far more difficult because it requires that people change their priorities, loyalties, beliefs, and habits[18]. Too often organizations mistake adaptive challenges for

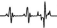

technical challenges and are surprised when the input of a technical expert fails to create the expected improvements.

Unlike technical change that can simply be mandated from above, adaptive change requires understanding and participation at the grassroots level and requires adaptive leadership[18]. Adaptive leaders have to orchestrate changes in culture and should employ many of the strategies described in the next chapter. Anytime there is adaptive change, there will be winners and losers, and those who stand to lose usually have all the political power. And that is why adaptive change is far more challenging than technical change.

Improvements in safety and quality will require profound changes in the way nurses, physicians, and patients interact, as well as a significant increase in their efforts to learn new approaches to improve quality and safety. Defenders of the status quo will become upset and will feel a sense of loss as their "tried-and-true" approaches to patient care are challenged. Because most of us do not understand adaptive change, we will become dissatisfied with the adaptive leader and call for his or her dismissal.

As Machiavelli observed five hundred years ago, adaptive leadership is dangerous and requires great courage. Ideally those with the greatest power within a health care system should be adaptive leaders. At minimum, adaptive leaders lower in the power structure must have strong support and understanding from the highest levels of the administration. Without this key condition, the adaptive leader is certain to fail and likely to be fired.

> **Key Points about Differentiating Technical from Adaptive Change**
> - Technical changes can be made following input from expert consultants and mandated from the top down.
>
> - Adaptive change requires cultural change:
>   - Far more challenging to accomplish
>   - Requires grassroots support
>   - Results in losses by those supporting the status quo
>   - Dangerous and requires courage
>
> - Most changes in our health care system will require adaptive change.
>
> - Health care leaders need to be adaptive leaders.

Managing Disequilibrium

One of the most important tasks of an effective adaptive leader is to help others to manage the stresses of change. A useful analogy is the combustible automobile engine. As the engine produces power to move the car forward, it produces heat as a natural byproduct. The motor's temperature is controlled by its cooling system, and if the cooling system fails, the engine overheats and stalls. Similarly, an expected byproduct of adaptive change is disequilibrium, and the adaptive leader must act as the cooling system.

The adaptive leader and his/her leadership team should show compassion and empathy for those experiencing the discomfort of change, and they need to maintain disequilibrium within the productive zone (see gray region in **Figure 5.3**). This requires continual monitoring of those undergoing change and continual modifications of strategy. Keeping everyone in the productive zone of disequilibrium creates sufficient stress to mobilize people to focus and solve the problem they would prefer to avoid. Allowing disequilibrium to boil out of control will distract everyone from their ultimate goal, lead to destructive rebellion, and stall all progress.

One of the most common ways to avoid stress and slow change is by work avoidance[18]. As an example, let's look at what happened after the famous Supreme Court decision to desegregate our nation with "all deliberate speed." The Southern states delayed implementation for decades by utilizing political filibustering, claims of financial hardship, as well as public protests[19]. The task of solving the problem of segregation was avoided, and the disequilibrium caused by the Supreme Court decision was dissipated (dashed line, **Figure 5.3**).

A second method for avoiding change is to discredit the adaptive leader. When Kathleen Long attempted to change the educational requirements for professional nurses, she experienced a strong emotional response by a fellow nursing leader who favored the status quo (see **Case 5.6**). This nurse leader was hoping to block further change and reduce disequilibrium by discrediting Dr. Long (dashed line, **Figure 5.3**).

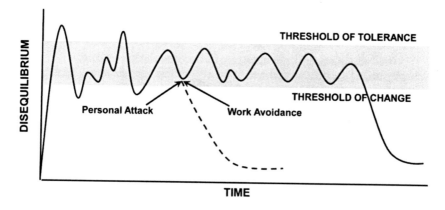

Figure 5.3. Maintaining a productive zone of disequilibrium (see text for details, adapted from Heifetz et al.[18])

If desegregation had been quickly and effectively implemented in the South, and a four-year degree for registered nurses immediately mandated, over time the attitudes of whites in the Southern states and resistant nursing educators would have changed, and these changes would have been accepted as the new status quo. Upon achieving a new status quo, equilibrium can be reestablished (disequilibrium near zero, far right solid curve, **Figure 5.3**).

Key Points about Managing Disequilibrium
- Adaptive changes always generate disequilibrium.
  - There must be anxiety and a sense of loss to bring about meaningful changes in attitudes and the ways of doing things.

- Adaptive leaders must
  - show compassion and understanding to those experiencing change and
  - monitor closely the extent of disequilibrium and maintain it within the productive zone.

- Leaders should be aware of avoidance behaviors:
  - Work avoidance, failing to implement the changes
  - Attacking the credibility of the adaptive leader

- Once the adaptive change has been implemented, disequilibrium will dissipate, and the change will become the status quo.

Designing Effective Interventions

Just like any effective organizer, the effective adaptive leader develops a carefully constructed strategy, and many of the key elements of designing effective strategies and tactics are covered in the next chapter. Just like any other organizer, adaptive leaders begin with one-on-one meetings to recruit allies and create a leadership team. He or she properly frames the planned adaptive change by employing personal narrative. As described later, when developing the strategy for intervention, it is important to determine the ripeness of the situation. What is the sense of urgency? Are caregivers and administrators ready to attack the situation?

As in all life, the devil is in the details. Everyone agrees on the overall importance of improving safety and quality. After all, who could be against these initiatives? However, when an adaptive leader begins to identify specific issues such as rounding inefficiency, many will claim that the specific system identified for improvement is not broken and does not require change. As

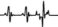
noted above, specific changes cause discomfort and result in loss. And when it comes to adaptive changes, if there is "no pain" there is "no gain."

The leadership team can be very helpful for determining whether the disequilibrium of a specific change can be managed. In some instances the pain will be too great, and the initiative will have to be delayed or modified. For example, rather than completely desegregating all communities and all schools, the first adaptive change utilized by federal officials was to desegregate the schools by bussing students.

When designing change, effective adaptive leaders examine where they fit into the overall organizational picture. They understand how they are viewed by other groups and subgroups and how comfortable they were with the leader's prior leadership roles. Whenever possible, experienced adaptive leaders ask guiding questions to help those who will be affected by the change to better understand the rationale and to allow them to assist in designing the intervention.

Once the intervention has started, the effective adaptive leader holds steady, remembering that the improvement is no longer his or hers, but theirs. He or she allows them to adapt the preliminary plan. The leader remains present and whenever possible silently monitors the group's progress because these observations will provide helpful data for modifying future strategy. A supportive and empathetic approach reduces disequilibrium and positions the adaptive leader as an ally. Patience and poise allow the leader to weather the predictable effects of cultural change.

As the initiative moves forward, the adaptive leader watches who becomes actively involved and who takes on the new ideas as their own, and he or she notes who resists the new ideas. The different factions can be mapped and their viewpoints detailed. The improvement initiative is often framed in different ways for different factions. For example, a rounding system improvement described in Chapter 4 could be framed as a way of increasing respect and communication for the nurses, as a way of saving time for the residents and the senior physician, and as a way of improving the educational experience for the medical students.

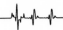

Finally, while monitoring the improvement group's actions, effective adaptive leaders anticipate and counter avoidance tactics. Avoidance is a normal human behavior and is to be expected during adaptive change. Issues of disloyalty, loss, and fear of incompetency will always accompany meaningful change, and people naturally desire to avoid these issues. As discussed above, one of the most aggressive methods for disrupting an improvement project is to employ personal attacks that often focus on the motives of the adaptive leader. By recognizing this tactic, and by returning the focus to the work that needs to be done, leaders can usually deflect such attacks. High-level administrators need to recognize this tactic for what it really represents: a mechanism for reducing the anxiety of adaptive change.

Key Points about Designing Effective Interventions

- Utilize organizing techniques, including one-on-one meetings, to recruit allies, a leadership team, and perform careful strategic planning.

- Carefully manage disequilibrium, and when it's too high, step back and change the strategy.

- Hold steady and allow others to take ownership and adapt the intervention.

- Anticipate and counter avoidance tactics.

- Expect personal attacks and deflect them by focusing on the intended goals.

- Enlist the support and encourage the understanding of high-level administrators.

Effective Adaptive Leaders Avoid Common Traps

The world is filled with adaptive leaders who have crashed and burned because they fell into common traps. And I have to confess that I have inadvertently fallen into nearly all of these traps during my career. Being aware of what not to do can help all adaptive leaders to remain effective leaders of meaningful change[18].

Effective adaptive leaders…

- …don't lose their perspective. The passion of the cause and single-minded devotion to bringing about an improvement can narrow one's perspective. An adaptive leader can become dangerously single minded and fail to make adaptive midcourse strategic changes. During my efforts to improve work rounds at our institution (see Chapter 4), I lost perspective and ignored the complaints of fellow faculty members. I now realize that opposing voices should be regarded as canaries in a coal mine and should be regarded as helpful feedback.

- …don't become self-righteous. Excessive certainty about the cause has the potential to trigger strong resistance in others. Being overly strident can take away the ownership of others and can make them feel they are being forced to change. Effective leaders try to "pull by persuasion" and never push those below them to change. Experienced adaptive leaders accept the reality that change will be slow. I have to confess that while trying to encourage others to adopt an improved inpatient rounding system, I became impatient, insisted on the rightness of my initiative, and tried to push it on others.

- …don't become the chief purpose officer. Effective leaders realize that reminding the group or organization of the larger purpose behind the improvement project is important. However, they also exercise restraint. When an adaptive leader infuses the same purpose into every meeting, others quickly discount his or her voice, and this leader will become marginalized and ineffective. I now realize that is exactly how fellow faculty members reacted to me. In every conversation I would bring up the importance of teamwork in health care. In retrospect, I had ignored the upward stares and wrinkled foreheads that were providing nonverbal warnings of their frustration with my continued proselytizing.

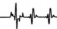

- ...don't become martyrs. Experienced adaptive leaders recognize that their activities will generate tension, and they develop strategies to reduce excessive tension. Excessive disequilibrium will cause concern on the part of higher-level administrators and can lead to the adaptive leader's professional death. When the heat gets excessive, it is important to step back and modify the strategy by designing smaller steps to advance change. When a leader is removed from the campaign, all his or her hard work is likely to have little or no effect, and the effort will have been wasted.

Key Points about Common Traps
- Don't lose perspective and become single-minded.

- Don't become self-righteous.

- Don't become the chief purpose officer.

- Don't be a martyr.

When Possible, Inspire

Emotions are major drivers of action, and adaptive leaders should practice personal narrative and stories of the suffering of individual patients to inspire caregivers to improve how they care for patients. Mary's case represents such a personal story, and her story is intended to touch the heart to encourage the head and hands to act. Some nurses and many physicians fear that emotions will interfere with their ability to make objective decisions. And all caregivers do need to recognize and appropriately manage personal emotions in order to prevent depression, anger, and burnout. Appropriate emotional control allows caregivers to effectively treat each patient[20]. However, when it comes to inspiring meaningful change, the sharing of emotions should be encouraged. When a particular story touches your heart and you become tearful, don't stop. Instead, talk through the emotions, understanding that by opening up to the audience, you will create trust and a sense of genuine sharing. When speaking about a difficult problem, pause and allow your audience to reflect on the challenge. The tone and volume of a speaker's voice can also be effectively used. A loud trumpeting voice can signal an important concept, and a softer, graceful pace can sooth and calm the audience.

The telling of personal stories is an effective start, but leaders of change also need to listen with their hearts. They need to listen with compassion and curiosity to the concerns of those trying to implement changes on the front lines. Reflective listening that includes comments like "I understand," "I see," and "That must have been hard" frame the adaptive leader as an ally, as someone who is trying to fix things, not tear them down. Too often adaptive leaders "go down with their mouths open."[18] People rarely get taken down because they spent too much time listening.

Key Points about Inspiration
- Utilize variations in voice tone, loudness, and pace.
- Embrace emotions, and keep talking through the tears.
- Also listen from the heart:
  - Listen with compassion and curiosity.
  - Make reflective statements.

Balance Your Life

Taking on the role of being an adaptive leader at any level in an organization has the potential to become all-consuming. Each of us must be aware of the downside of devoting too much time and energy to one activity. As outlined above, this approach has the potential to become counterproductive. The best antidote against burnout is to create purposeful balance by allotting sufficient time and energy to our other spheres of life. The importance of family and friends cannot be overemphasized. Too often leaders with great potential neglect their families, and the resulting unhappiness eventually bleeds over

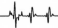

to their work. Interests related to church, synagogue, or mosque; community outreach; outdoor activities; and sports should also be nurtured. These venues allow each of us to invest in other interests and reduce our dependence on work for our fulfillment.

Adaptive leaders also require one or more close colleagues outside of the organization with whom they can share their concerns and obtain advice. A confidant can mirror your ideas and can provide frank and honest feedback. Wives or husbands are often very effective in this role, and it is no coincidence that leaders so often publically acknowledge the support of their spouses. Finally, in addition to attending to their emotional health, adaptive leaders should schedule sufficient sleep and exercise, as well as adhere to a healthy diet to ensure that they maintain the physical and mental energy required to bring about meaningful change.

Key Points about a Balanced Life
- Schedule sufficient time for your family.
- Have interests outside of work that are personally rewarding.
- Recruit one or more close colleagues outside of work as a confident.
- Get sufficient sleep and exercise, and adhere to a healthy diet to maintain your energy.

Conclusions

As health care undergoes transformational change over the next decade, leadership will be of critical importance. Leadership will be required not only in the executive suites but also on the front lines and at every level—from janitors, to ward clerks, to social workers, and on up to nurses, physicians, and administrators. Effective leadership can be taught, and among the most important skills to be learned are time management, priority setting, self-recognition of each leader's potential unique contributions, the ability to focus on strengths, and most importantly, the ability to make well-informed

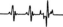

decisions that lead to action. Leaders should be courageous and have strong core values, as well as openness, modesty, and a sincere interest in others. Most importantly of all, health care leaders need to orchestrate adaptive change. Without adaptive leaders who are willing to manage cultural change and endure the strident resistance of those protecting the status quo, our health care system will never undergo the sustained and continual improvement our patients deserve.

References

1. M.B. Balik, and J.A. Gilbert. 2010. *The Heart of Leadership*. Chicago, IL: Health Forum, Inc.

2. Nitin Nohria, and Rakesh Khurana. 2010. *Handbook of leadership theory and practice : an HBS centennial colloquium on advancing leadership*. Boston, Mass.: Harvard Business Press.

3. M.D. Cohen, and J.G March. 1974. *Leadership and Ambiguity: The American College President*. New York, NY: McGraw-Hill.

4. J. Antonakis, A.T. Cianciolo, and R.J. Sternberg, eds. 2004. *The Nature of Leadership*. London, UK: Sage Publications Inc.

5. R. Wageman, D.A. Nunes, J.A. Burruss, and J.R. Hackman. 2008. *Senior Leadership Teams*. Boston, MA: Harvard Business School Press.

6. William Shakespeare, and John Ward. 1676. *The tragedy of Hamlet Prince of Denmark : as it is now acted at his Highness the Duke of York's Theatre*. London: Printed by Andr. Clark, for J. Martyn, and H. Herringman .

7. James C. Collins. 2001. *Good to great : why some companies make the leap-- and others don't*. 1st ed. New York, NY: HarperBusiness.

8. Bill George, and Peter Sims. 2007. *True north : discover your authentic leadership*. 1st. ed, *The Warren Bennis signature series*. San Francisco, CA: Jossey-Bass.

9. D. Carnegie. 1981. *How to win friends and influence people*. New York, NY: Pocket Books.

10. F.D. Loop. 2009. *Leadership and Medicine*. Gulf Breeze, FL: Fire Starter Publishing.

11. J. Ciulla. 2004. Ethics and Leadership Effectiveness. In *The Nature of Leadership*, edited by J. Antonakis, A.T. Cianciolo and R.J. Sternberg. London, UK: Sage Publications, Inc.

12. Peter F. Drucker. 2006. *The effective executive*. New York: Collins.

13. J. Wooden, and S. Jamison. 2005. *Wooden on Leadership*. New York, NY: McGraw-Hill.

14. J. Cohen. 2007. *Sick*. New York, N.Y.: Harper Collins Publishers.

15. Leonard L. Berry, and Kent D. Seltman. 2008. *Management lessons from Mayo Clinic : inside one of the world's most admired service organizations*. New York: McGraw-Hill.

16. J.D. Waldman, F. Kelly, S. Arora, and H.L. Smith. 2004. The Shocking Cost of Turnover in Health Care. *Health Care Management Review* January-March:1-7.

17. Rose Rivers. 2011. Personal observations.

18. Ronald A. Heifetz, Alexander Grashow, and Martin Linsky. 2009. *The practice of adaptive leadership : tools and tactics for changing your organization and the world*. Boston, Mass.: Harvard Business Press.

19. C.J Ogletree. 2004. *All Deliberate Speed*. New York, NY: W.W.Norton & Company, Inc.

20. D. E. Meier, A. L. Back, and R. S. Morrison. 2001. The inner life of physicians and care of the seriously ill. *JAMA* 286 (23):3007-3014.

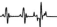

Chapter 5 Exercises

1. What leadership role can you take in health care?

    a. As a nurse is there any area in your system where you could influence fellow workers to make an improvement?

    b. What would be your strategy for change?

2. How efficiently do you use your time?

    a. Keep a log for twenty-four hours, and review how your time was spent.

    b. Is the majority of your time spent focusing on patient care?

    c. What activities are distracting you from this primary focus?

3. What are your strengths and weaknesses? How can you maximize your strengths to further your nursing leadership goals?

4. How do you make decisions?

    a. Do you carefully look from all possible points of view?

    b. How well do you investigate the facts before deciding?

    c. Based on your reading, are there any changes you plan to make in how you make effective decisions?

5. Are you an adaptive leader? Why or why not? Are there adaptive changes that need to be made in your nursing school or workplace?

6. Have you ever experienced strong opposition after proposing or attempting to bring about a change in the way things are done or a change in attitude? Describe your experiences.

7. Would you do things differently after reading this chapter?

–6–

CULTURE IS NOTHING MORE THAN GROUP HABIT

How Could Changes in Medical Culture Have Improved Mary's Care?

Guiding Questions

1. Who was Samuel Adams, and what can he teach us about changing the culture of our health care system?

2. Who should be our primary constituencies and why?

3. Why are one-on-one meetings important?

4. What do we mean by the story of self, the story of us, and the story of now?

5. Why do we need specific measurable goals, and how do we create them?

6. What is the difference between a strategy and tactic?

7. How do we ensure action?

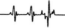

Lost Opportunities

Now what kind of an attitude is that, "these things happen?" They only happen because this whole country is just full of people who, when these things happen, they just say "these things happen," and that's why they happen! We gotta have control of what happens to us.

—*Ethel Merman in* It's a Mad, Mad, Mad, Mad World (*to see the video go to* http://www.youtube.com/watch?v=ou1hODlpseY, *accessed 2/5/11*)

At the time of Mary's illness, the academic medical center where she was cared for had a weak safety culture, one in which there was poor teamwork, poor communication, little coordination of care, poor supervision of trainees, and little evidence of institutional learning[1]. I never received any official apology or acknowledgement of the errors that had accompanied Mary's care. A cone of silence surrounded these events. As a junior faculty member, I was fearful of speaking out and only did so after leaving the institution. When I discussed Mary's case with colleagues soon after her hospital discharge, fellow academic physicians responded, "That's the way it is," "These things happen," and "Mary's illness was one in a million. She was just unlucky." Were my expectations unrealistic? We all must keep in mind that retrospective critiques are fraught with assumptions. But as outlined in Chapters 2 and 3, when errors occur, all caregivers, patients, and patient families need to ask why and to learn from a thorough analysis of each mistake. This approach represents one of the first steps toward creating a culture of safety[1].

Mary's illness was complicated and extremely rare. And such challenging cases test a health system and its culture. The care that Mary received in the early stages of her illness can only be characterized as fragmented and at times impersonal. And I was an insider. I can only speculate on the treatment an outsider might have received under the same circumstances. In Mary's case, the system failed and exposed a physician-focused culture where the care of patients was of secondary importance as compared to both research and family obligations.

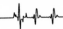

Over the past decade, the institution where Mary received her care has fully embraced the principles of safety and quality. It has initiated programs to improve organization accountability, to improve coordination and transitions of care, and to reduce variations in practice. In fact, it's become one of the leaders in health care systems and quality improvement, and the probability of Mary's case recurring in this facility now is extremely low.

How Can Organizing Help?

How can we bring about cultural change in our health care systems? How do we overcome the natural tendency to accept what is? When we simply shrug our shoulders and say "These things happen," we are promoting unnecessary suffering and death in our hospitals and clinics. In the words of Ethel Mermen, "We gotta have control of what happens to us."

When it comes to the profound cultural changes required to improve our health care systems, top-down mandates promise to induce push-back and anger and are unlikely to be effective. Sustainable cultural change requires grassroots organizing, and this approach has the potential to create consensus and improve morale. Organizing techniques can greatly enhance the ability of health care leaders at every level to change their culture and empower their organizations to participate in the continual improvement of patient care. Effective organizing can allow leaders to create power with rather than power over[2]. Most excitingly, organizing can greatly increase the leadership quotient of an institution and render that institution more nimble in its ability to adapt to the many challenges of our evolving health care systems. In fact, as the criteria for insurance payment shifts from quantity to quality, the skills required to organize health care providers may prove to be among the most fundamental of skills required for institutional survival.

These techniques can be used to transform the culture of a single floor, a care unit, a division, a department, a specific group of employees or patients, as well as an entire hospital or entire health system. These methods can and should be used whenever people need to be mobilized to accomplish specific goals, particularly when those goals represent changes in the way things are done. And as outlined in the preceding chapters, there are a huge number of changes required to transform health care delivery. When anyone speaks about organizing, most people immediately think of unions and political campaigns; however, as will be discussed in this chapter, these same methods can and should be used to transform patient care in our hospitals and clinics.

One American colonist, Samuel Adams, organized what should be regarded as the most effective campaign in history. This remarkable Founding Father won over nearly every colonist in Massachusetts and changed the course of history. And just as a cultural change was the first step toward the United States' independence from the British, a change in culture can serve as the first step in curing the ills of our present health care delivery system.

The Story of Samuel Adams, Organizer of the American Revolution

Samuel Adams forged a profound change among his fellow countrymen that led to the American Revolution and the birth of democracy. The specific strategies and tactics he developed more than two hundred years ago have subsequently been used by Caesar Chavez and the farm workers to defeat the powerful California grape growers[3], Martin Luther King to overcome segregation[4], and by the Obama campaign to defeat the seemingly unstoppable presidential front-runner, Hilary Clinton[5]. American history is a story of change and renewal, and many of the major transformations in the United States have come about as a consequence of organizers who were capable of harnessing the power of people to achieve shared goals in the face of uncertainty.

Why is Samuel Adams Not Appreciated?

In his speech on July 4, 1976, the two hundredth celebration of the Declaration of Independence, President Gerald Ford highlighted four Founding Fathers—John Adams, John Hancock, Thomas Jefferson, and Benjamin Franklin—as having played central roles in bringing about our independence. In reality, Samuel Adams was the key figure that orchestrated a fifteen-year campaign from 1758–1773 against the repressive rule of the British that led to the Continental Congress and the Declaration of Independence (see **Figure 6.1**). He remains to this day one of the least appreciated of the Founding Fathers. Why?

The answer to this question reveals two of the fundamental characteristics of effective and transformational organizers. Samuel Adams recruited and empowered others to bring about change. He eschewed personal fame and fortune. He did not want the public to focus on him but rather to focus on the ideas and principles that subsequently led to our independence.

Second, because he was an adaptive leader who favored change, those who favored the status quo vilified him. The Governor of Massachusetts called him "The Chief Incendiary." The opposition suggested he was encouraging rule by "mobs" and blamed him for all violent acts by the colonists. However, in reality these acts were based on a spontaneous groundswell of anger toward British taxation and restrictions of freedom. As a consequence of the British and the American British Loyalists' negative propaganda, many historians have mischaracterized Samuel Adams as an irresponsible troublemaker when in reality, as acknowledged by many of his fellow patriots, he was the central and guiding force behind American independence.

What Events Explain Samuel Adams's Opposition to the British?

Samuel Adams was the Founding Father that first recognized the dangers of Great Britain's progressive financial stranglehold on the American colonies. Personal misfortune sensitized him to the oppressive nature of British rule. Soon after Samuel completed Harvard College, his father suffered financial ruin as a consequence of a capricious ruling by the British Parliament. The Parliament outlawed his father's Land Bank and mandated that he be liable for all bank debts.

At the time of his father's bankruptcy, nearly all colonists were content under the rule of the British. The colonies were growing and prospering, and few recognized the potential impact and meaning of British taxation. In the 1760s the British began enforcing the taxation of molasses and subsequently

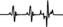

added the Sugar Act that taxed sugar, followed by the Stamp Act that taxed all legal documents, and the Townsend Act that taxed paint, paper, glass, and tea. When Samuel Adams complained to Benjamin Franklin, he retorted that fighting British taxation was tantamount to "hindering the sun's setting."

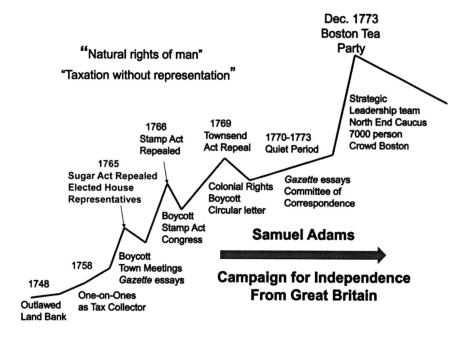

Figure 6.1. Time line for Samuel Adams's campaign for American independence. The horizontal axis is time. The vertical axis represents the degree of campaign activity. By December of 1773, Samuel Adams had successfully harnessed the personal power of the Massachusetts colonists to seek independence from Great Britain. Shortly thereafter, the other twelve colonies also embraced the goal of independence.

How did Samuel Adams Campaign against British "Financial Tyranny"?

Samuel Adams employed four fundamental approaches to change the attitudes of his fellow colonists toward the British. He persistently employed each of the techniques, often simultaneously, to convert the colonists from complacent British subjects to independent Americans willing to risk their lives to achieve the freedom to determine their own future.

1. One-on-One Meetings and Formation of a Leadership Team

His primary strategy at the beginning of his campaign in the mid-1750s was one-on-one meetings and the creation of a leadership team (see **Figure 6.1**). As an elected tax collector, he came into direct contact with men from all walks of life. Using one-on-one meetings, he shared his high aspirations for the Massachusetts Bay Colony on the docks and in the taverns, markets, shipyards, shops, stables, streets, and squares of Boston. He met with his younger second cousin John Adams and urged him to become involved in civic affairs. Initially John helped Samuel, but after several years he withdrew from politics, only to return after the Boston Tea Party. Samuel also recruited young and influential physicians and lawyers and merchants, including John Hancock. Through the long-standing political organization the Caucus Club, he formed a leadership group. This important group discussed the goals of their campaign and formulated the strategies for publicizing the dangers of British rule.

2. Personal Narrative

He utilized the power of the pen and his oratory to capture the emotions of the colonists and create a sense of urgency. Joining with others, he purchased a newspaper, *The Public Advertiser*, and also became an active contributor to the *Boston Gazette*. Under various pseudonyms he wrote essays espousing the natural rights of men and the concept of taxation without representation. He created a strong vocabulary of campaign phrases and fundamental ideas about human rights and governance that subsequently formed the basis for our Declaration of Independence. In public meetings he was renowned for his passionate fire-and-brimstone speeches. During his fifteen-year campaign, he used personal narrative to touch the hearts of nearly every Massachusetts Bay Colony member and transformed the colonists from apathetic and complacent British subjects to independent Americans who demanded the freedom and the right to determine their own destiny.

3. Public Meetings and Uniting of Organizations for a Single Purpose

He organized large public meetings and was an active member of many civic organizations. He brought together large crowds in Faneuil Hall, Old

South Church, and under a large elm tree that became known as the Liberty Tree. At the time of the Boston Tea Party, a crowd of seven thousand gathered in Boston from all of the nearby towns. This represented nearly half the population of the city at that time. Despite his tremor and rather frail appearance, his searing blue eyes, remarkable energy, and inspiring oratory proved very effective at motivating his audience to take action.

4. Crafting of Strategy and Encouraging Action

Working with his leadership group he crafted innovative strategies to overcome the many obstructions created by the British government. When the British levied the Sugar Act, it was Adams who proposed that merchants agree not to import British goods in order to create financial pressure to rescind this tax. He called this action "nonimportation." John Hancock and other merchants lost money as consequence of these actions, and many including Hancock withdrew from Adams's campaign. One hundred years later this strategy became known as a boycott, and to this day remains a common pressure tactic to bring about change. When the governor suspended the Massachusetts House of Representatives, Samuel Adams organized a large town meeting that included delegates from ninety-eight towns and eight districts.

In order to create greater power, he worked to unite the thirteen colonies in support of a common cause by organizing Committees of Correspondence in every town and colony. These letter-writing committees shared their concerns and developed strategies for countering the British desire for financial and political dominance. He turned negative events into sources of energy and resistance. After British soldiers shot five colonists for throwing snowballs, it was Samuel Adams who labeled this sad event a "massacre" and encouraged the wide distribution of Paul Revere's famous Boston Massacre engraving.

The highpoint of Samuel Adams's carefully orchestrated campaign strategy came in 1773 during the standoff over three ships docked in Boston Harbor waiting to unload British tea (**Figure 6.1**). He organized the North End Caucus, where representatives from Boston and the outlying towns unanimously agreed that British tea could not be unloaded to the docks of the Boston Harbor. When the ships arrived, the captains honored the colonist's

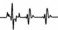

wishes. However, British law declared that all goods had to be unloaded within twenty days of the initial docking.

As the twentieth day arrived, the captain went to the governor to request that he be allowed to sail back to Great Britain without unloading his tea. The governor refused. The captain returned to a huge crowd gathered in protest. It was clear to all that the British would unload the tea in the morning. Should Adams publically agree to a violent riot? He had consistently opposed such actions and had consistently encouraged the strict use of civil disobedience. The inciting of crowd violence would brand him a traitor and a criminal. As the huge crowd waited impatiently, he called out, "This meeting can do nothing more to save the country" and disbanded the crowd.

As if on signal, a group of forty men in Indian disguises immediately yelled out "Boston Harbor a tea-pot tonight!" As the delighted crowd watched, the "Indians" rushed to the ships and with their hatchets, broke apart all three hundred and forty-two tea chests and dumped them into the harbor. The Boston Tea Party galvanized nearly all colonists in support of independence

from Great Britain. This event precipitated a British blockade of Boston Harbor and the landing of four British troop regiments. The Battle of Lexington and Concord, the convening of the Continental Congress, the Declaration of Independence, and the Revolutionary War soon followed[6-9].

GATEWAY

http://bit.ly/s9umll

Key Points about Samuel Adams
- He was the older second cousin of John Adams and the Founding Father primarily responsible for the American Revolution.

- His father suffered financial ruin as a consequence of an unfair treatment by the British Parliament.

- He waged a fifteen-year campaign to urge the apathetic colonists to rebel against the financial tyranny of the British.

- He waged his campaign utilizing four key elements:
  1. One-on-one meetings to recruit leadership teams
  2. Personal narrative through newspaper essays, posters, and fire-and-brimstone speeches
  3. Strategy and tactics that included boycotts, large town meetings, and the formation of new organizations including the Sons of Liberty and the Correspondence Committees
  4. Action in the form of protests and unanimous policy agreements culminating in the ultimate action, the Boston Tea Party—an action that led to the American Revolution

Basic Principles of Organizing

The story of Samuel Adams provides great lessons for transforming the American health care system. Just as he overcame apathy utilizing effective campaign strategies, health care providers can achieve this same important goal. However, those of us who choose to organize others to improve the culture of health care, beware. Just like the great Founding Father of our country Samuel Adams, we too may be misunderstood and vilified by those who want our systems to remain the same. When we suggest that conditions in our health care systems are not ideal, "Remember human beings do not like to look square in the face of tragedy. Gloom is not popular and we prefer the 'out of sight out of mind' escape"[10] (see tactics on page 271 on how to avoid gloom).

To bring about true change, organizers need to use the many tactics and skills employed by great leaders like Samuel Adams. Just like Samuel Adams, they must be patient and "start from where the world is… not where you would like it to be."[11] Any reader hoping to construct a campaign needs to realize that simply reading this chapter will not make you an effective organizer. Organizing is a practice that you primarily learn by doing (see the exercises at the end of the chapter).

As the famous Danish philosopher Kierkegaard described:

> Imagine a pilot, and assume that he had passed every examination with distinction, but that he had not as yet been at sea. Imagine him in a storm; he knows everything he ought to do, but he has not known before how terror grips the sea farer when the stars are lost in the blackness of night; he has not known the sense of impotence that comes when the pilot sees the wheel in his hand become a plaything for the waves; he has not known how the blood rushes to the head when one tries to make calculations at such a moment; in short, he has had no conception of the change that takes place in the knower when he has to apply his knowledge[12].

Case 6.1. To improve how patients are treated at a university health care system, the administration kicked off a campaign to encourage all employees to focus on the needs of patients. A stage was set up in the atrium of the hospital, and the CEO of the system, the dean of the College of Medicine, the director of the hospital, and the director of nursing all spoke. Each speaker made a promise about how they would personally improve patient care. More than three hundred people crowded the hospital atrium, and each person signed up for an oval blue button with white lettering saying, *I Promise*. Many nurses, clerks, and receptionists signed the volunteer sheet. Over the next two weeks the nurse volunteers organized the nurses on each ward to create a collage that included everyone's written promise. On one ward, the nurses posted a huge paper sunflower. Each petal contained one nurse's promise for how he or she would personally improve each patient's experience. All the nurses proudly wore *I Promise* buttons. It was clear that nearly every nurse in the hospital had embraced the campaign.

Effective campaigners must first ask the question: I am organizing *who* to do *what?* In **Case 6.1**, the administration was organizing all employees interacting with patients to focus on the needs of their patients and patient families. Once a goal has been established, the organizer must touch the heart (personal narrative) to gain the attention of the head (strategy and tactics) to encourage and guide the hands (action). In **Case 6.1**, each administrator made a personal promise that touched the hearts of the audience.

http://bit.ly/uWNzMn

Before beginning a campaign, it is critical to identify and understand your constituency—that is, those you plan to organize. Hospital nurses assisted in organizing the campaign and knew their fellow nurses well. They participated in multiple one-on-one encounters to recruit nurse champions for each ward. Organizing cannot take place in a distant office but, as exemplified by the nurses working in the *I Promise* campaign, must take place on the front lines.

Once one-on-one meetings have recruited four to five like-minded individuals, a leadership team can be formed to create measurable campaign goals. The nurses working on the *I Promise* campaign formed a leadership team that came up with the idea to encourage each hospital ward to create a collage containing the nurses' personal promises. Their campaign goal was to have a nursing *I Promise* collage on every ward within two months. Upon creating this goal, the team generated strategies and tactics to achieve it. Using additional one-on-one meetings, they identified an *I Promise* nursing champion for each ward, and each ward champion recruited three to four nurses to join their *I Promise* ward leadership team.

The ward campaign team divided up the entire roster of nurses on the floor and quickly took action. Within two weeks they had personally contacted every nurse to write and post their promise. The nursing campaign successfully achieved its goal. Within two months every ward had a nursing *I Promise* collage. Upon completion of their first *I Promise* campaign goal, the nursing team held a grand celebration in the hospital auditorium where congratulations posters decorated the walls, and they tallied the actual number of individual promises for each ward. A special luncheon was served to all participants as a reward. These nursing campaign teams have remained active and are presently creating new campaign goals for the next six months as they continue their campaign to improve the experience of each patient within their health system.

Key General Points about Organizing

- Be patient. "Start from where the world is… not where you would like it to be."

- Organizing has to be learned by doing.

- First ask the question, "I am organizing *who* to do *what?*"

- Understand your environment and your constituency before beginning your campaign.

- Understand the three faces of power:
  ○ The overt power of the board room and administrators
  ○ The more subtle power of the ability to control the agenda
  ○ The ability to convince the have-nots that they deserve to lose, and to foster apathy

---

The Three Faces of Power

Before introducing you to the major constituencies of the health care system, you must first understand the three "faces" of power utilized to maintain the status quo[13]. The first and most apparent face of power is seen in the boardroom. This can be quickly be determined by observing who wins the policy battles and who has the most influence on hospital and personnel decisions. These overtly powerful individuals and boards vary from hospital system to hospital system. However, before designing a campaign strategy, it is critical that the organizer understands and appropriately addresses the first face of power.

The second face of power is the ability to decide who sits at the table and to control what is included on the agenda. Those in power can prevent issues from being acted upon by never allowing them to be considered by committees empowered to take action and also by excluding "troublemakers" from their deliberative bodies. In the 1950s and early 1960s, our U.S. Congress frequently employed this gatekeeper strategy to block desegregation.

The third and least appreciated face of power is the creation of apathy among the have-nots. When the allocation of any valued resource is determined, there will be winners and losers. Under conditions where there is a disparity of resources and power, the winners claim they deserved to win and convince the losers that they deserved to lose. When discussing the withdrawal of financial resources from those who were disabled and in need, Reverend William Sloan Coffin noted that the wealthy and well-off had convinced our politicians that the "needy are greedy and greedy are needy."[14]

Constituencies in the Health Care System

Armed with an understanding of the three faces of power, you now can better understand the interrelationships between the constituencies within the health care system. Our health care system has several important constituencies that often don't appreciate their mutual interests. And this fragmentation is a critical condition that has contributed to lack of meaningful change over the last decade, despite the overwhelming evidence that our systems are failing our patients.

Patients

The most important constituency and the one we should all be focusing on is the patient. However, sadly, as a consequence of our current payment system, our patients have little power over what happens to them. The insurance company is supplying what the patient needs—health insurance—and previously the insurance company could threaten to drop any patient from their insurance pool. Patients usually do not have a large number of insurance choices, and furthermore, it is often difficult for patients to differentiate between the qualities of the different insurance plans. Thus the patient-insurance relationship is asymmetric and the insurance company has most of the power. The U.S. health care reform bill signed into law in 2010 promises to improve these conditions and empower the patient.

In addition to the insurance company-patient relationship, there is the patient-doctor relationship. Because the insurance company pays the physician for the services provided to the patient, a true customer-supplier relationship between the patient and the doctor does not exist. Because patients are not directly paying for the physician's services, they have little interest or control over how the physician manages their health care. Furthermore, the patient usually has little medical knowledge and therefore must trust that the physician is doing what is most cost effective and is designing treatment plans that are truly in the patient's best interest. Thus the patient-doctor relationship is also asymmetric, with the doctor possessing most of the power. Furthermore, both insurance companies and physicians have convinced patients that they are receiving the "best" medical care. Thus these two major stakeholders have successfully utilized the third face of power by creating patient apathy. These conditions are correctable as outlined in the final chapter and make patients an ideal constituency for future organizing to bring about the needed changes in our health care system.

Physicians

The second major constituency is the physician. The majority of physicians chose their profession because they wanted to cure and comfort the sick. However, changes in our health care system have caused an inadvertent shift in physician perspective and mission. The complexity of health care has increased, and health care has become more procedure- and test-based. The reimbursement system has increasingly rewarded quantity over the quality of care. The patient too often is seen as a vehicle for the billing of tests and procedures. To compound this problem, physicians graduate from medical school with high educational loan burdens, necessitating that they choose the more lucrative procedural-based over the cognitively-based specialties.

As previously discussed, there is a wide geographic disparity in health care expenditures in the United States, and the lack of a positive correlation between expenditures and quality indicates that more expensive care and more procedures do not translate into better health and better outcomes. To control the continued rise in expenditures, insurance companies are increasingly attempting to micromanage physicians, forcing them to play the "mother may I" game (i.e., procedures and hospital visits must be preapproved by the insurance companies). This condition has reduced the power of the physician to make decisions and to manage their practices. Furthermore, payments for procedures and for volume rather than for the quality and effectiveness of care have progressively undermined the altruistic spirit of many doctors and weakened the doctor-patient relationship. These conditions have led to physician discontent and make physicians prime candidates for the campaign to improve our health care system.

Nurses, Nurse Practitioners, and Physician Assistants

The third major constituency is nurses, nurse practitioners, and physician assistants. In nearly all systems, these individuals are paid a fixed annual salary (performance bonuses may be provided in some instances). As a consequence, unlike physicians and insurance companies, these health care providers do not have the same inherent conflict of interest.

Nursing standards dictate the number of inpatients one nurse should care for, eliminating the pressure to increase the volume of care. The nurse-patient relationship remains intact, and with the exception of salary disputes and work rules, this constituency is among the most stable and constant. They continue to serve the altruistic role they envisioned when they began their training. Because the nursing supply remains limited, when dissatisfied, they can readily move to a more positive and supportive environment. Nurses tend to be well organized and have maintained their power within the health care system. In my view, nurses remain the true defenders of high-quality care for patients, and physicians should emulate the networking and team approaches embraced by nursing. Given their networking capabilities and values that align with the needs of our patients, nurses have the potential to be the primary leaders in the campaign to improve our health care delivery systems.

Students

A fourth constituency and the constituency that has the greatest potential to support change is our students. Nursing students, medical students, and those studying to be physician assistants have less of a stake in the status quo. They are capable of more objectively evaluating our systems, and as historians and sociologists have repeatedly observed, it is the young who most often serve as the catalyst for change. They have the energy and creativity, and lack the family and financial obligations that too often lead to apathy toward or fear of system reforms. Student campaigns also teach our students about leadership and teamwork—two vital skills for improving our health care systems.

There are a number of other constituencies with a potential to be organized, including ward clerks, other office personnel, technicians, hospital maintenance employees, and transporters. And depending on the goals of the campaign, they may also possess the resources and energy to bring about change.

Who is most open to change?

When focusing on any constituency, it is important to keep in mind that not all members of a constituency will be open to innovation and change. Studies of the diffusion of innovation reveal there are five behavioral categories (**Figure 6.2**)[15]. First there are the early innovators—the creative few who are constantly developing innovations. The next group consists of the early adopters—those who are excited about change and are eager to try new innovations. A third group is the early majority—individuals who are more deliberate in their decision to embrace change. Campaigns should focus on these three groups, particularly the early adaptors and early majority.

Too often organizers misdirect their focus on those who are more resistant to change, the skeptics and the traditionalists (also called laggards). Experience

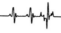
shows that these groups only embrace change after the early adaptors and the early majority have proven the efficacy of the innovations, and they have become an accepted practice. Traditionalists are the most resistant to change and only accept change after the innovation is mandated by a governing body. Focusing on skeptics and traditionalists usually proves counterproductive and often leads to frustration and hardening of resistance.

Key Points about the Major Constituencies of Health Care

- Patients are the most important constituency; however, they lack power and have asymmetric relationships with insurance companies and physicians. They continue to blindly accept the U.S. system as the "best in the world."

- Physicians have progressively increased their focus on moneymaking procedures and tests. The quantity and volume of care are the predominant measures of success. The original patient-centered focus has deteriorated.

- Nurses, nurse practitioners, physician assistants continue to focus on the needs of patients, are well organized, and continue to fulfill their original mission as true patient advocates.

- Students do not have the financial and family obligations of the more senior members of the system. They promise to be the primary vehicle for change.

- You need to remember Rogers's innovation diffusion curve and focus your attention on the early adopters and the early majority.

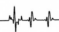

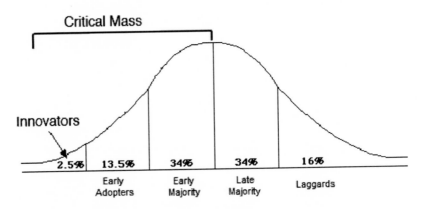

Figure 6.2. Roger's innovation diffusion curve, from Rogers EM. Diffusion of Innovations, New York, NY: Free Press; 2003

One-on-One Meetings

Connecting with others through one-on-one meetings is a fundamental skill that is required to initiate any campaign. Samuel Adams was extremely effective at one-on-one meetings, and in his role as a tax collector, he was able to share his ideas and visions with others and learn of their concerns and aspirations. When their goals and interests proved mutual, he recruited them to one of his many leadership groups and encouraged their active participation in the campaign for American independence. Nelson Mandela, the first postapartheid president of South Africa, provides another dramatic example of the power of one-on-one meetings. Nelson Mandela was confined to jail for twenty-seven years because of his opposition to apartheid. Rather than becoming bitter and withdrawn, he constantly met with fellow political prisoners and shared his vision for multiracial governance. He taught through his one-on-one meetings, and as a consequence the jail where he was imprisoned was nicknamed "Mandela University." Thanks to his very large network of political friends and allies created while in prison, upon his release in 1990, Nelson Mandela was able to guide the Afrikaner National Party in negotiations to establish a multiracial government. During his four years as president of South Africa, his powerful personal network proved invaluable

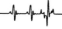

for establishing the foundations for tolerance and for creating a consensus for basic reforms[16].

Few people anywhere at any time achieve the stature of Samuel Adams or Nelson Mandela. However, we can all become effective one-on-one campaigners. Those who care for patients have already been taught and practice one-on-one interactions, and these skills are fundamental for creating the ideal patient-health care provider relationship. In all effective interpersonal relationships, each person must be willing to share something that the other person values. This exchange can only take place if the person initiating the interaction first attracts the other person's interest. Calling someone by his or her first name and showing genuine interest in the other person are among the most effective ways of accomplishing this goal[17].

Once both people are attentive, an exploratory phase can begin. This critical phase serves to establish mutual trust and creates emotional as well as intellectual connections. The two-way sharing of personal details about one's life and life choices is not only helpful for establishing trust but also for determining shared interests. What were your life's crucibles, and how did you overcome them? These stories tell us about how the individual deals with adversity, and they are likely to predict how a person will react to the uncertainties that commonly arise during campaigns. They also serve to inspire and to instruct (see the personal narrative below). To be effective in one-on-one interactions you must be an effective questioner. Questions draw out the individual, and the phrasing and tone of your questions allow you to demonstrate empathy and true interest. Finally, as your first conversation comes to a close, you must determine if there is a basis for a relationship. If there is, then you both must commit to meet again.

One-on-one interactions must always be honest and forthright, and from the very start it is important to inform the other person that you are interested in recruiting him or her to join you in a campaign. Personal relationships within a campaign should be relatively loose in nature. These relatively weak relationships create less confining interpersonal bonds that result in stronger action-oriented campaign organizations. One-on-one meetings can take as little as ten to fifteen minutes. They are often invigorating and enjoyable because sharing of stories with others is a fundamental activity of humans, who are by nature very social animals. These activities will not only lay the foundations for your campaign, but they will also improve your interpersonal skills.

Key Points about One-on-One Meetings
- One-on-one meetings are the underpinning of all effective campaigns.

- They consist of sharing of something of value from each individual.

- An effective one-on-one meeting has three phases:
  - Greeting—need to gain the other person's attention
  - Exploratory phase—sharing of personal experiences and values through effective exploratory questions
  - Commitment—agreeing on mutual interests and shared goals and deciding to continue the relationship by arranging a second meeting

- Relationships need to be loose and should not be confining in order to allow the formation of effective action-oriented organizations.

Personal Narrative: The Story of Self, the Story of Us, and the Story of Now (Heart)

There are three basic components in all campaigns: heart, head, and hands. Personal narrative is about heart, about creating emotions that motivate the listener to become involved. Effective personal narrative has been the hallmark of many of our most revered orators, including Martin Luther King, Robert Kennedy, Ronald Regan, and Barack Obama. Each of these orators knew how to effectively touch the heart, and each inspired listeners to take action.

The Importance of Emotions

Why are emotions important, and where do they arise? For man, particularly when placed in threatening situations, emotions are critical for survival. Fear and anger stimulate the fight-or-flight response, resulting in the production of adrenaline and noradrenaline, and the release of these hormones increases our alertness and ability to quickly respond to danger. These responses arise primarily in the limbic system, found at the base of the brain, between the cerebral cortex and the brain stem[18]. This region is critical for the processing of stimuli including sound, vision, and touch. Emotions are generated in multiple regions of the brain. One of the most important regions is the amygdala, and this structure is extensively connected to the prefrontal cortex, the region of the brain just beneath the forehead that is responsible for decision making[19]. Damage to the amygdala markedly impairs the ability to synthesize information and make choices[20]. Our recent understanding of neurophysiology emphasizes the importance of emotion in changing opinion and stimulating us to act, and effective personal narrative arouses feelings and encourages our audience to take action.

Key Points about Emotions
- Are a key warning signal in times of danger

- Encourage action

- Result in rapid and often permanent learning

- Arise in the limbic system
  - Amygdala one primary site
  - Strong connections with the prefrontal cortex where decisions are processed

- Allow us to decide and create urgency and action

The Story of Self

There are three components of personal narrative that should be combined to motivate goal-directed commitment: a story of *self*, a story of *us*, and a story of *now*. In most effective narratives, the story of *self* leads seamlessly into the story of *us*, followed by the story of *now*.

A story of self explains why you have been called to serve. Many of you

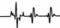

have had a personal experience related to a dramatic and frightening illness or a frustrating encounter with a health care provider or system. If properly described through effective personal narrative, these stories can touch the heart of the listener and provide strong motivation for change. All effective narratives require three basic elements: an unexpected challenge, a choice, and an outcome.

In the case of medical illness, as exemplified by Mary's story, the patient and her family encounter unexpected challenges when they enter the health care system. Sadly, too often those of us required to use this system are called upon to adapt or work around the many obstacles we encounter. In describing these events, we must offer personal details of how we coped with uncertainty and challenge. We need to create a moment where the listener can enter. Such stories usually describe needless pain and suffering, and like Mary's story, they too often end in a near-death experience, or a serious injury.

When effectively described, these stories can arouse deep emotion. They can warn the listener of the dangers they and their families may encounter if they are unlucky enough to require medical care. Effective stories of self can motivate the listener to act and to join with the storyteller in a campaign to improve a specific problem in our health care system. Narrating a story of self takes practice and repeated rehearsal. Through diligent practice, each of us can progressively improve our ability to personally touch the heart of our listener. I have told Mary's story over and over in speeches to motivate physicians to improve our systems of care, and my hope is that my full description of Mary's story in the first chapter has captured your heart and will motivate you to take action.

The Story of Us

The story of *us* relates our personal stories to the conditions in our entire communities. This story should describe why we as a community need to act and why our group has the capacity to bring about change. In the case of health care, statistics about deaths caused by preventable errors, general experiences related to lack of access to care, dramatic differences in the cost of care in different geographic regions, and overall surveys of quality can all serve to motivate your community to action. As described above, each health

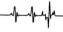
care constituency has unique perspectives and skills to bring about change, and these can be highlighted in your story of us. What are our shared aspirations, values, and commitments? In the case of health care providers, our common and very strong desire to improve the health and well-being of our patients should serve as a central theme. A quote that I personally return to again and again is, "The secret of the care of the patient is *caring* for the patient," by Dr. Francis Peabody of Boston City Hospital, 1927[21]. All caregivers should identify with this important piece of advice.

The Story of Now

The story of *now* describes an urgent specific condition that we as a group can correct or improve. The speaker needs to challenge the audience to take action by joining the campaign. The goal of the campaign needs to be focused and outcomes must be measurable. Also the goal must have a meaningful impact and specifically address the problem or problems described in the story of self and the story of us.

In **Case 6.1**, the kickoff of the campaign primarily focused on the story of now by emphasizing the need to enhance the patient experience at the university health center. In all likelihood, the story of now would have been more compelling if it had been preceded by a story of self and a story of us. Let's look at another urgent health care problem: hospital-acquired infections. Despite the fact that hand washing remains the most effective action we can take as health care providers to prevent the spread of disease-causing bacteria, in many hospitals there is no sense of urgency or emotional commitment to hand washing. How could we address this important problem? First describe the plight of an individual patient (story of self) such as Ginny's story, which is available on YouTube video http://www.youtube.com/watch?v=s5x1f3_NJX8 (accessed 2/5/11).

In 1996, Ginny had just returned from a delightful vacation in Las Vegas, where she had enjoyed skydiving. On her return to Boston, she slipped off a curb and broke her ankle. She had expected a full recovery; however, surgical repair of her fracture was complicated by methicillin-resistant *Staphylococcus aureus* (MRSA) *osteomyelitis* contracted in the hospital. Treatment of her infection was delayed, and despite many courses of antibiotics and twenty-eight surgeries over the next five years, her infection spread, necessitating a life-saving leg amputation.

During her illness she also suffered three respiratory arrests and became blind in her right eye as a consequence of an infected right retinal artery. As she closed the narrative of the video showing her downward spiral and eventual recovery, she concluded, "Anyone can break an ankle, but that is where the story should end."

Key Points about Personal Narrative

- Personal narratives have three components:
  - Story of self—a personal story with three elements: an unexpected challenge, a choice, and an outcome; critical that it evoke emotion and motivate the listener

  - Story of us—must closely relate to the story of self and describe a general condition in the community that requires change; emphasizes why the community needs to act and why the audience has the capacity to bring about change

  - Story of now—describes a specific goal and specific actions related to the story of self and the story of now; calls on members of the audience to join the organization to achieve the specific goal

- All three elements need to be seamlessly linked.

- Speakers should avoid fixed scripts because personal narrative is iterative and adapts to the audience and prevailing conditions.

Nearly everyone watching this video will experience deep emotions that should encourage them to act by always washing their hands and by campaigning to improve hand washing compliance. We should follow Ginny's story by the story of us that outlines the overall frequency of hospital-acquired infections,

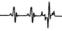

the resulting morbidity and mortality, and the cost to our health care system. The story of us should then be followed by an urgent call to join a hand washing campaign in the hospital with the goal of 100 percent compliance within three months (story of now).

A well-crafted personal narrative has a far greater likelihood of motivating health care providers than sending email requests, creating a web-based educational program, giving a dry informational lecture, or placing posters on the doors. The creation of a personal narrative is an iterative process, and it will change over time depending on the audience, prevailing attitude, and current conditions. The speaker should avoid a fixed script and allow the narrative to evolve and improve over time as he or she becomes a more skilled and perceptive narrator.

Leadership Teams

Effective campaigns should never be about a single leader. The charismatic lone hero takes the limelight from others and quickly burns out trying to manage the day-to-day complexities of an active campaign. Just as Samuel Adams empowered other leaders to achieve the goal of independence from Great Britain, those organizing campaigns to improve health care must empower others to lead and organize. "Leadership is accepting responsibility to create conditions that enable others to achieve purpose in the face of uncertainty."[22] A true leader recruits and trains new leaders, and these leaders in turn recruit and train additional leaders, progressively increasing the leadership quotient and human resources. Unlike financial campaign resources that become depleted, effective campaigns progressively increase their human capital over time.

Samuel Adams created leadership teams throughout his fifteen-year campaign. Historical documents do not fully describe how he identified potential leaders or recruited them; however, it is likely that, through one-on-one meetings in his role as a tax collector and subsequently as a member of the House of Representatives, he was able to identify talented young men with the organizational skills, drive, and proper values, who subsequently became good leaders. Two of his recruits, John Adams and John Hancock, became active members of the Continental Congress and along with him signed the Declaration

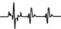

of Independence. Subsequently John Adams served as the second president of the United States. Clearly Samuel Adams had a good eye for potential leaders.

Choosing the Ideal Recruits for the Leadership Group and Campaign

Similar to Samuel Adams, as a health care provider you will come in contact with large numbers of fellow providers, and you too will need to identify potential leaders for your campaign. The essential components of leadership in health care were fully described in the previous chapter. However, there are certain characteristics that will be helpful for the initial selection of your campaign leadership team. Leadership is informally practiced throughout the health care system, and many of these leaders are not those who have official positions but rather individuals who take the initiative when they encounter unexpected problems. In addition to having initiative, organizers should show empathy and be good listeners that understand the needs of their fellow providers and patients. They should be curious, imaginative, and open to change. A sense of humor is also helpful, combined with large dose of humility and a healthy ego. Arrogance should be avoided because arrogance often leads to conflict within the leadership team, and it usually reflects a poor self-image. Finally, courage and resilience are valuable traits because uncertainty and the unexpected are commonly encountered during effective campaigns for change.

Managing New Recruits

Once potential leaders have been identified, they need to be recruited to leadership roles, initially through one-on-one encounters and then by providing each recruit with leadership opportunities within the campaign. Opportunities should not be simple tasks but rather responsibilities for achieving a specific goal. For example, rather than assigning recruits to email or phone a specific number of health care providers to join the campaign organization, they should each be assigned the responsibility for recruiting five health care providers to the next organization meeting, empowering each recruit to create their own methods for accomplishing this goal. This serves as an initial leadership test, and during this trial period it will be important for the organizer to be available to provide advice and coaching. Coaches must avoid inadvertently taking over the new recruits' work. Ideally they should show interest in their activities and serve as mentors. By creating small tests of leadership, one can quickly determine who can be counted on and who has earned a place on the leadership team. In voluntary campaigns, leadership depends on interdependence and collaboration. A power-over-leadership dynamic should be avoided in favor of a power-with-leadership model. Because voluntary campaigns do not pay participants, organizers must persuade, not command.

Managing the Leadership Team

After the leadership team has formed, the team must be launched. The key components of an effective launch as well as the management of ongoing team dynamics were covered earlier, and all organizers will need to be familiar with these principles in order to create an effective team. A critical daily task is to ask the leadership team, "What are we doing well, and what could we improve?" This reflective question allows members of the leadership to team to air their positive and negative impressions and allows the team to constantly improve.

One of the most important initial tasks of the campaign leadership team will be to decide on the specific goal or goals for your campaign. This is often a difficult task, and many leadership teams break apart at this juncture because of strong differences of opinion and an inability to achieve compromise or consensus.

Key characteristics of effective campaign goals are: 1) the goals must be closely linked to the personal narrative and clearly relate to the emotional forces and values that motivate the leadership team; 2) the outcomes of the team's goals must be measurable in order to determine the progress and success of the campaign; and 3) the goals should neither be so narrow that they have minimal impact nor too broad rendering them impossible to achieve.

For example the goal of convincing two physicians to communicate more effectively with nurses will have a minimal impact on how a hospital functions, while the goal of improving physician-nurse communication throughout the U.S. health system would be overly ambitious. A realistic goal might be to enhance physician-nurse communication on one hospital floor over six months and monitor communication through nursing, physician, and patient survey questionnaires before, midway, and at the completion of the campaign.

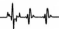

Key Points about Leadership Teams
- A highly functional leadership team is a critical component of any effective campaign.

- Leadership is accepting responsibility to create conditions that enable others to achieve purpose in the face of uncertainty.

- Leadership
  - ○ should not be about holding on to power as the lone wolf or single hero but
  - ○ Should be about empowering everyone to take on leadership responsibility.

- You should identify and recruit potential leaders who possess
  - ○ initiative;
  - ○ good empathic listening skills;
  - ○ curiosity, imagination, and openness to change; and
  - ○ humility, a healthy ego, courage, and resilience.

- You should manage recruits by
  - ○ providing them with the responsibility to achieve a specific meaningful goal that requires creativity and leadership and
  - ○ coaching them, without taking over their work, asking guiding questions, and providing performance feedback.

- Launch your team and manage team dynamics (see Chapter 4) and repeatedly ask the leadership team, "What are we doing well, and what could we improve?"

- Together, create the goals for the campaign. The goals:
  - ○ Must be closely linked to the personal narrative.
  - ○ Consist of measurable outcomes.
  - ○ Have the proper scope: not too narrow, providing minimal impact, and not too broad, making them impossible to achieve.

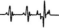

Strategy

Samuel Adams proved to be a brilliant strategist who outmaneuvered the British at every turn. He utilized a talented and diverse leadership team to formulate and discuss different strategic alternatives and to create contingency plans based on different possible outcomes. Many of the twists and turns of his campaign were unexpected, and changes in strategy were often developed on the fly.

What Is Strategy?

Strategy provides the means to convert "what you have" into "what you need" to get "what you want."[2] Strategy turns resources into power. In nearly all campaigns there is an initial power imbalance, and this imbalance can be corrected in one of two ways: increase resources (people and/or money) or create conditions that allow resources to be used more effectively. In health care, the latter strategy will in most situations be the preferred approach. For example, if the goal is to convince health care providers to wash their hands when coming into each new patient's room, one strategy would be to ask the administration to pay for observers on every floor to monitor hand washing. An alternative strategy would be to empower the bedside nurses to insist that all health care providers entering their patients' rooms wash their hands. Nurses could be trained on how to engage in constructive dialogue to encourage adherence. The latter approach leverages an established resource (the bedside nurse) to solve a serious problem (the spread of hospital-acquired bacteria from patient to patient).

Strategy and Tactics During the Campaign

Strategy is a game plan. Organizers are very much like athletic coaches. Before each football game, the offensive coach creates a game plan based on the strengths and weakness of his and the opposing team. Each individual play is a tactic, and the sequence of the plays and specific plays chosen represent the strategy or game plan. Just as the coach must have an intimate knowledge of each of his player's strengths and weaknesses, the organizer must be able to evaluate accurately the campaign's resources and potential constraints.

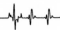

Often the coach decides on the first four to five plays before the start of the game, and these plays are designed to probe the weaknesses of the opposition. Based on the outcomes of the initial plays or tactics, the game plan or strategy will often need to be modified. Good strategy needs to be flexible and creates contingencies for what "to do when the impossible happens."[23] The football coach may decide that plays over the left side of the line will be most effective; similarly the organizer may decide to target one administrator, one floor, or one clinic to achieve the intended goal. In sports, life, and campaigns, timing is also critical. "Timing is to tactics what it is to everything in life—the difference between success and failure."[11] Delays in implementing specific tactics can result in a loss of motivation and momentum.

Moving too quickly without allowing key individuals to accept the initial changes created by your campaign can result in resistance and jeopardize the desired outcome (create excessive disequilibrium as described in the previous chapter). Periodic thoughtful reflection is critical to properly crafting strategy. Just as the offensive coach sits high above the field, observing the game, organizers need to periodically step back and review their successes and failures and alter their strategies based on these reflections. Finally, when creating strategy, it is important to always keep in mind the ultimate goal. In the case of health care, the goal should always be patient-centered, efficient, high-quality, error-free care.

Campaign Time Lines

As shown in **Figures 6.1** and **6.3**, campaigns are best visualized as a linear time line. Each campaign goes through different phases. Initially a foundation must be created. This entails one-on-one meetings, recruitment of a leadership team, and developing a rich understanding of the resources, environment, and culture. In the cases of Samuel Adams and Nelson Mandela, the development of a foundation took years. In the case of health care, because those who will be organizing will usually be insiders who work within the system, the achievement of a solid foundation promises to be more efficient. The formal beginning of the campaign is announced by a kickoff. This is generally a large public gathering where the campaign is announced and the leadership team is introduced (see **Case 6.1**). Personal narrative plays a critical role at these

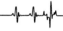

events to motivate the attendees to join the campaign. The setting of a specific date for the kickoff creates a sense of urgency and a deadline for the leadership team. This deadline forces the leadership team not just to plan but to act. At the completion of the kickoff it is critical that those in the audience be requested to make a commitment by signing up for a specific committee, agreeing to attend a subsequent meeting, or agreeing to help with specific task. In **Case 6.1**, everyone who received an *I Promise* button and signed a sheet providing contact information.

Key Points about Strategy

- Strategy converts "what you have" into "what you need" to get "what you want." Strategy turns resources into power, and power can be increased in two ways:
  - Increasing the resources—increase personal capital and/or increase financial capital.
  - Leveraging the resources you have—create conditions that allow you to use your resources more effectively.

- Strategy is a game plan, and tactics are the individual plays or actions within the game plan.

- Strategy requires
  - an accurate assessment of the campaign's strengths and weakness and its resources and constraints;
  - flexibility and contingency plans for the inevitable what-ifs;
  - careful timing;
  - periodic thoughtful reflection; and
  - continual focus on the ultimate goal—patient-centered care.

- The strategic time line is best viewed as a linear line with peaks and valleys of activity:
  - Begins with a quiet building phase, primarily one-on-one meetings
  - Announces the campaign publically by a kickoff
  - Designs multiple small peaks to recruit additional resources

---

Several smaller peaks of activity such as a luncheon event, a group educational session, or a rally designed to recruit new leaders and new participants usually follow the kickoff. The goal of each peak is to increase human resources and capacity. The minipeaks lead up to a final peak where the maximum number of constituents has been mobilized to achieve the specific goal. The final peak is generally an exciting event and represents the culmination of weeks to months of recruiting, planning, and action. In many cases, the peak for a quality improvement campaign will be the achievement of a measurable milestone, such as a 90 percent reduction in medication errors or 99 percent hand washing adherence. The peak will celebrate a major accomplishment (see **Case 6.2**). Finally the peak is followed by resolution. In the case of health care quality, this would be reflected as a sustained quality performance measure.

Strategy in Health Care Campaigns

Given the complexity of the health care system, strategic planning promises to be challenging. The leadership team must fully explore the power structure and be familiar with the personal attributes and attitudes of the administrators responsible for the activity or process that the campaign is hoping to improve. Health care systems suffer from extensive regulation and are mandated to achieve certain quality measures and milestones. These regulations do not always reflect the activities of those on the front lines and often are not embraced or understood by those directly caring for patients. These regulations render many administrators fearful of significant change because change has the potential to make conditions temporarily worse before they improve. Therefore, before launching any campaign to improve quality, it will be critical to first achieve alignment with the hospital administration. The majority of campaigns should be directed toward convincing frontline care providers to follow accepted and proven quality procedures and processes from highly regarded organizations dedicated to improving health care quality. Therefore, if the leadership team has properly introduced their campaign goals, the responsible administrator or administrators need to practice adaptive leadership and welcome these ground-up initiatives.

Campaigns to improve health outside of the hospital will not suffer the same formal administrative barriers. However, depending on the specific goals of the campaign, the leadership team will be tasked with trying to unite disparate organizations such as churches, other volunteer organizations, the public health department, the hospital systems, public officials, primary care physicians, physician assistants, nurses, and most importantly the residents of the community. Understanding the local organizational structures, culture, and politics will require extensive one-on-one meetings with key community leaders, as well as the residents of the community. Leadership team members will also have to meet with the leadership bodies of the community and government organizations.

Key Points about Strategy in Health Care System Campaigns
- Hospital and clinic-based campaigns
  - must achieve alignment with the administration;
  - should beware of extensive regulatory rules that foster resistance to change;
  - should target their primary constituency: frontline health care providers; and
  - should set their primary goal at convincing providers to embrace proven practices that improve patient care quality, efficiency, and safety.

- Community based campaigns
  - must achieve alignment of multiple voluntary community organizations, government and private health care organizations, and public officials;
  - should beware of organizational rivalries and silos;
  - should target their primary constituency: the people of the town, county, or region; and
  - should set their primary goal at convincing the community organizations to embrace the concept of a healthy community by creating systems that encourage healthy behavior.

Only after this groundwork has been completed can an effective prelimi-

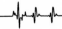

nary campaign strategy be designed. The leadership team must be cognizant of organizational rivalries and silos. By appealing to common shared goals and by utilizing personal narrative, many of these potential conflicts can be overcome. These approaches can be used not only in local communities in the United States, but also can be employed to empower those living in developing countries to bring about needed changes in their villages, towns, and cities to improve health.

Action

Too often leadership teams continue to plan and argue about specific strategies rather than acting. An effective campaign requires participants to jump into the water rather than tiptoe around the shoreline. But how does an organization encourage action?

Securing Commitments

First and foremost the organizers need to secure commitment to build human capital. Securing commitments is difficult for many of us because we fear rejection. When we ask the question, "Can I count on you?" the person can say, yes, maybe, or no. When we hear a yes, we are pleased and rewarded, but we need to realize that follow-up by repeated phone calls is mandatory. You must remind the newly committed of their upcoming commitment several days before the scheduled commitment and most importantly within twenty-four hours of the commitment to meet or participate in an activity. Personal reminders are critical for ensuring a yes is truly converted into an action. The most dreaded reply is maybe because there is neither a commitment nor a refusal. Such contacts will need further one-on-one meetings to clarify their potential commitment.

Many of us naturally take a no personally, failing to realize this is a common occurrence when organizing. In the African American voter registration campaign in the early 1960s, campaign organizers described doors being slammed in their faces or, even more frightening, guns pointed at them. However, the most effective canvassers came back again and again, eventually softening resistance and gaining trust[24]. Fortunately, most campaigns for health care quality and health will not be met with such negative reactions. Organizers can view one-on-one recruiting like a fishing trip. The fisherman baits the hook and waits for the fish to bite. Sometimes the fish ignores the bait, other times it will nibble, and every now and then it will bite. Fishermen rarely take the lack of interest by the fish personally; they simply change the bait to make it more appealing to the fish. That is exactly what the effective organizer must do.

Many fellow health care providers, patients, and patient families will provide excuses for why they do not want to become involved. One common reply is likely to be, "This is the way it is, and it will never change no matter what I do." To address this valid concern, the potential recruit must be convinced that "you can make a difference" (YCMD). It is important when discussing our health care system to first point out the remarkable successes modern medicine has achieved. Dramatic reductions in mortality and morbidity due to myocardial infarction, stroke, and cancer represent exciting successes and suggest that if health care providers and patients focus on the problems of health care delivery, similar dramatic improvements in the processes of care can be achieved. When discussing the problems with our health care system, the organizer must be careful not to paint too negative a picture, or potential participants will become overwhelmed by gloom and doom and will develop the impression that the problems are too large for any one person to make a difference. Emphasize the key point that many small steps eventually lead to a large step or advance.

A second common reply may be "Our health care system is excellent. I have not seen these errors you keep talking about." The story of us and the story of now should answer this second objection. By creating a sense of urgency concerning the high incidence of errors and needless deaths, the stories of self and us are likely to overcome such apathy toward change.

Probably the most common reply will be, "Sorry, but I simply don't have time." Time is a precious commodity for everyone, and effective campaigns respect time by being highly organized with regards to meeting agendas and task assignments. One effective response is to promise that the campaign will make effective use of the participant's valuable time. Suggest that the recruit participate in one event, and if dissatisfied, he or she is welcome to withdraw. When a potential recruit actively participates, commitment naturally increases. By providing an escape clause in a personal contract, the perception of being strong-armed is reduced.

Creating Measurable Goals, Monitoring Progress, and Creating Meaningful Work

Once a critical mass of campaigners has been recruited, the group must develop a series of measurable outcomes designed to achieve the goals. Clear measurable outcomes allow the group to assess its progress. Each outcome should be accompanied by a specific deadline, and when that deadline is achieved, the group success should be celebrated. Measurable outcomes also allow the team to determine which individuals are succeeding, as well as who is failing. The group can share the best practices of those who are succeeding and learn from the mistakes of those who are failing.

Coaching through directive questions is integral to this process, and the learning derived from small successes and failures steadily increases the team's tactical skills. Events and people need to be carefully coordinated by encouraging time lines and creating milestones. When possible, charts should be created documenting the progress of the campaign to provide visual sense of accomplishment. One of the most critical elements of action is the design, assignment, and assessment of specific tasks. Ideally all tasks should be meaningful and serve to increase motivation, commitment, and leadership capacity.

Once an action plan has been designed, the leadership team needs be assured that the three criteria for an effective action plan have been fulfilled. The plan should solve the problem and achieve the goal or goals of the campaign. Secondly, the action plan should strengthen the organization by increasing understanding, building relationship commitment, and generating new resources. Thirdly, it should facilitate the growth of the individuals who participate in the action plan[25].

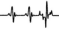

Key Points about Action
- The single most important action is securing commitments:
  - A yes requires phone follow-up to convert a yes into true action. Provide an escape clause so the recruit does not feel strong-armed.
  - A maybe requires additional one-on-one meetings.
  - A no should not lead to a sense of failure. Have the attitude of a fisherman and don't take a no personally.

- You should create measurable goals and monitor progress:
  - Learn from those who are succeeding and share their successes.
  - Learn from those who are failing and coach them on practices that have allowed others in the campaign to succeed.
  - Create milestones, and when possible use wall charts to monitor progress.

- You should create meaningful tasks that encourage volunteers to participate, learn, and grow.

- The action plan should
  - solve the problem and achieve the goal of the campaign;
  - strengthen the organization; and
  - facilitate the growth of the individuals who participate.

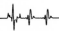

Case 6.2. As a college student at Harvard, Joe McCannon attended a course on organizing. His professor challenged the entire class to "make a difference in the world." After graduation, this challenge lingered in the recesses of his brain. Several years after graduation, Joe decided to join the Institute of Health Improvement (IHI) because he strongly identified with their goal to improve patient safety. However, progress in reducing errors and preventing deaths in the United States was slow. And in the spring of 2003, leaders of IHI reasoned, "Why not organize a national campaign to accelerate change?" Joe was chosen as the campaign manager, and he began applying the lessons he had learned in his organizing class. He quickly created a core leadership team and assigned specific responsibilities to each member.

The campaign kickoff (see **Figure 6.3**) came at the IHI national meeting with a speech by the IHI President and CEO Dr. Don Berwick on December 14, 2004:

> I'm losing my patience. So here is what I think we should do. I think we should save one hundred thousand lives. And I think we should do that by June 14, 2006—eighteen months from today. Some is not a number; soon is not a time. Here's the number: one hundred thousand. Here's the time: June 14, 2006—9:00 a.m.

To touch the hearts of their constituency, the personal narratives of patients and patients' families who had suffered injuries or lost a loved one due to preventable hospital errors were shared with frontline health care providers, and the providers shared their own difficult stories. Utilizing group call-ins (many with over eight hundred callers), group emails, and electronic campaign newsletters, they were able to share and celebrate campaign progress. Most important, they traveled to the sites—in some months hosting as many thirty local learning events in states and systems across the country.

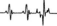

Through weekly meetings, Joe's leadership team adapted their strategy based on data provided by the district leadership teams. His team constantly reflected on their performance by asking, "What was going well, and what could be improved?" At the midpoint of their campaign, the leadership team organized a bus tour that traveled from Boston to Washington, D.C. and then across the entire United States, ending in Seattle, Washington (see **Figure 6.4 and 6.5**). They made stops at hospitals whose safety records exceeded their peers and celebrated their success with local health care

providers and administrators. These personal encounters energized both the IHI leadership and the local communities and provided a great boost to the campaign. On June 14, 2006, Don Berwick described the outcome of the campaign in a speech and press release:

> Hospitals enrolled in the 100,000 Lives Campaign have collectively prevented an estimated 122,300 avoidable deaths and, as importantly, have begun to institutionalize new standards of care that will continue to save lives and improve health outcomes into the future[26].

Their original goal was to sign up 1,600 hospitals; however, by the completion of their campaign they had succeeded in engaging 3,100 hospitals, representing approximately 75 percent of all hospital beds. By any measure the 100,000 Lives Campaign was a remarkable success[26].

Conclusions

Change has the potential to create conflict and can result in backlash when a single individual or even a high-level administrator serves as the primary driving force. Those who wish to bring about cultural change must begin with one-on-one meetings to recruit a leadership team, utilize personal narrative to attract like-minded followers, and create effective strategies and tactics to bring about action. The organizing techniques described in this chapter promise to be highly effective for achieving change on the front lines. As you complete this chapter, many of you may be thinking, *How can one person like me make a difference?* All of us need to keep in mind the lessons of Samuel Adams. Just as this resilient and persistent Founding Father organized an entire city, an entire region, and eventually all thirteen colonies to participate in the American Revolution, you too have the power to organize a revolution in health care.

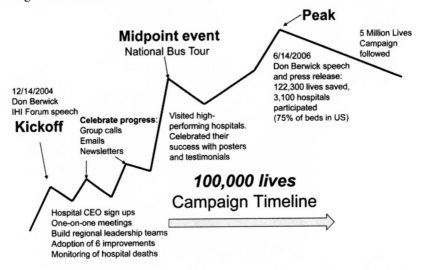

Figure 6.3. Institute of Health Improvement (IHI) 100,000 Lives Campaign. See **Figure 6.1** for further explanation of campaign time lines.

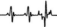

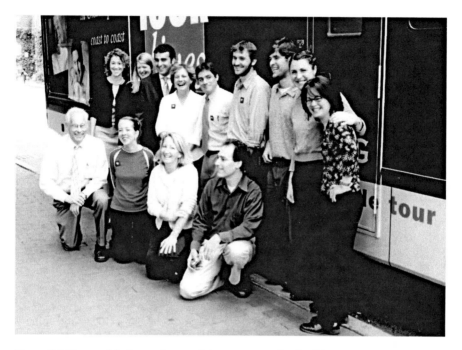

Figure 6.4 Picture of the bus and some of the participants for the IHI 100,000 Lives Campaign

100,000 Lives Campaign Bus Tour

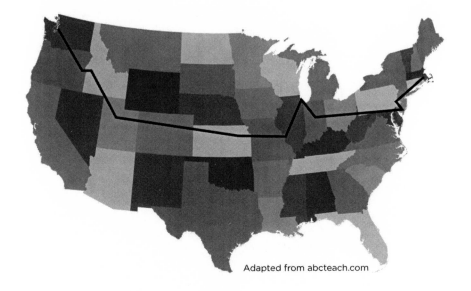

Adapted from abcteach.com

Figure 6.5. Map showing the route of IHI 100,000 Lives fifteen-city bus tour

References

1. A. Frankel, M. Leonard, T. Simmonds, C. Haraden, and K.B. Vega. 2009. *The Essential Guide for Patient Safety Officers.* Oakbrook Terrace, IL: Joint Commission Resources, Inc.

2. M. Ganz. 2009. Strategy Resources and Power. In *Harvard Kennedy School of Government*, Organizing Notes. Cambridge, MA.

3. M. Ganz. 2009. *Why David Sometimes Wins: Leadership, Organization, and Strategy in the California Farm Worker Movement.* Oxford, Great Britain: Oxford University Press.

4. S.M Glisson. 2006. *The Human Tradition in the Civil Rights Movement.* Lanham, MD: Rowman & Littlefield.

5. J. Hellemann, and M. Halperin. 2010. *Game Change: Obama and the*

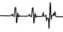
Clintons, McCain and Palin, and the Race of a Lifetime New York, NY: HarperCollins Publishers.

6. J.K. Alexander. 2002. Samuel Adams: *America's Revolutionary Politician.* New York, NY: Rowland & Littlefield Publishers, Inc.

7. R.V. Harlow. 1923. *Samuel Adams, promoter of the American revolution: a study in psychology and politics.* New York, NY: H. Holt and Co.

8. M. Puis. 2009. *Samuel Adams: Father of the American Revolution.* London, Great Britain: Palgrave Macmillan.

9. J.R. Galvin. 1976. *Three Men of Boston.* New York, NY: Thomas Y. Crowell Company.

10. S.D. Alinsky. 1974. *Reveille for Radicals.* New York, NY: Vintage Books.

11. S.D. Alinsky. 1971. *Rules for Radicals.* New York, NY: Vintage Books.

12. S. Kierkegaard. 1845. *Thoughts on Crucial Situations in Human Life; Three Discourses on Imagined Occasions.* Edited by Translated by David F. Swenson. Minneapolis, MN: Augsburg Publishing House.

13. J. Gaventa. 1982. *Power and Powerlessness: Quiescence and Rebellion in an Appalachian Valley.* Champaign, IL: University of Illinois Press.

14. W.S. Coffin. 1999. *The Heart is a Little to the Left.* Hanover, NH: University Press of New England.

15. E.M. Rogers. 2003. *Diffusion of Innovations.* New York, NY: Free Press.

16. R.C. Kanter. 2006. *Confidence: How Winning Streaks and Losing Streaks Begin and End.* New York, NY: Three Rivers Press.

17. D. Carnegie. 1981. *How to win friends and influence people.* New York, NY: Pocket Books.

18. D.A. Sousa. 2006. *How the Brain Learns.* Thousand Oaks, CA: Corwin Press.

19. C. D. Salzman, and S. Fusi. 2010. Emotion, cognition, and mental state representation in amygdala and prefrontal cortex. *Annu Rev Neurosci*

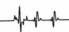

33:173-202.

20. A. N. Hampton, R. Adolphs, M. J. Tyszka, and J. P. O'doherty. 2007. Contributions of the amygdala to reward expectancy and choice signals in human prefrontal cortex. *Neuron* 55 (4):545-555.

21. F.W. Peabody. 1927. The Care of the Patient. *JAMA* 88:877-882.

22. M. Ganz. 2010. Leading Change. In *Handbook of Leadership Theory and Practice*, edited by N. Nohria and R. Khurana. Boston, MA: Harvard Business Press.

23. S. Kahn. 1982. *Organizing: A Guide for Grassroots Leaders*. New York, NY: McGraw-Hill.

24. C.M. Payne. 1995. *I've Got the Light of Freedom*. Los Angeles: University of California Press.

25. R. Hackman. 2002. *Leading Teams*. Cambridge, MA: Harvard Press.

26. C. J. Mccannon, M. W. Schall, D. R. Calkins, and A. G. Nazem. 2006. Saving 100,000 lives in US hospitals. *BMJ* 332 (7553):1328-1330.

Chapter 6 Exercises

1. What health care quality issues are you passionate about and why?

2. Pick a specific campaign project and create a measurable goal for your campaign.

3. Think of colleagues you would recruit through one-on-one meetings to join your campaign leadership team. Students should recruit fellow classmates to join their leadership teams.

4. Create an elevator speech (a two minute or less dialogue) that includes a story of self, a story of us, and a story of now.

5. Develop a strategy, taking into account those administratively responsible for the process you want to improve. Create a time line for your campaign.

6. Create an action plan and determine the milestones for achieving success. How will you know you have achieved your goal? This is an excellent class exercise for nursing students. Student groups can report on the narrative for their campaign, goals, strategies, and measurable outcomes.

–7–

BRINGING HOME THE RING

A Personal Five-Point Action Plan to Cure Health Care Delivery

Guiding Questions

1. Why are most of us so resistant to change?

2. How can I personally bring about changes to our systems of care?

3. How can I apply the lessons from the preceding chapters to ensure meaningful improvements in the quality, efficiency, and safety of patient care?

Together we have performed a very thorough root cause analysis of Mary's care. And we have explored how to apply our discoveries to the care of all patients. I know I speak for Mary and our children, Ashley and Peter, when I express the hope that Mary's close encounter with death will serve a higher purpose: to encourage each of us to actively participate in improving how all patients are cared for in our clinics and hospitals.

Immunity to Change

We have all read other books that call for action, and often we become temporarily inspired. We resolve to take action, only to lapse back into our usual routine. Too often our resolutions slip from our minds as we deal with the day-to-day issues that are part of living. To convert resolve into action will require fundamental changes in our behavior, and behavioral psychologists have known for decades that adults are creatures of habit who have great difficulty changing. Most of us are "immune to change."[1]

Many assume that adults over the age of thirty years can no longer change and learn that the adult's personality, views of the world, and approach to life are cast in stone. However, neuroscience has revealed that neural plasticity persists for life. The brain is able to continually remodel, to break down and create new synapses, new neural connections. What this means for the adult learner is that each of us can change and continually create new associations and new approaches to how we view and adapt to the world. As has been reiterated throughout this book, health care has become increasingly complex, and our old simplistic approaches are no longer effective. My hope is that after reading this book you now agree that our approaches to patient care must change. However, in order to bring about these changes, we as individuals will also need to change. We will need to literally reconfigure our brains to allow us to deal with the increased complexity of health care. We will need to correct what can be viewed as a brain and medical complexity mismatch[1].

Plan-do-study-act cycles can be effective not only for improving processes and structures within our hospitals, but they can also be used to improve ourselves. And just as we created primary and secondary driver diagrams to understand the underlying reasons for each dysfunctional medical process (see **Figure 3.6**), we can utilize these same methods to understand and correct our own deficiencies. When striving for personal change, the primary drivers are those things we do or fail to do that continually cause problems and interfere with our desire to achieve a new improvement goal or fulfill a new commitment. Secondary drivers are those hidden commitments that motivate the action or inaction that interferes with our ability to achieve our new goal.

As an example, let's assume you as a nurse are interested in improving patient care. You resolve to become an active participant on a hospital quality improvement team (see **Figure 7.1**). You are an inherently shy person, you are fearful of interacting with physicians, and you are a person who values getting along with others. These are your hidden commitments or the secondary drivers that will drive you to procrastinate in accepting the invitation to join the team, to fail to speak out at the meeting, and when you do speak, to avoid disagreements with others. All of these actions or inactions represent the primary drivers that will interfere with you becoming a member of the quality improvement team, sharing your perspective, and at times disagreeing with other team members.

GATEWAY

http://bit.ly/t6DVAM

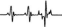

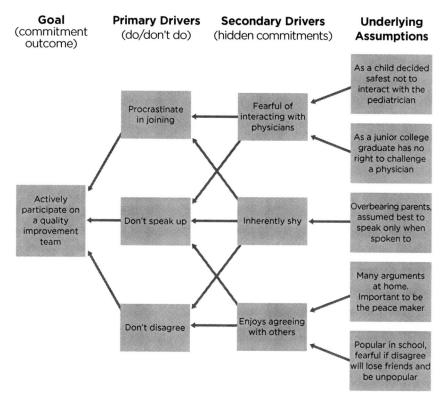

Figure 7.1. Immunity map for a nurse's participation on a quality improvement team.

Knowing your previous history and tendencies, you can predict your behaviors, but how can you change them? Many of us make New Year's resolutions to improve a personal or physical trait. But how often do we succeed? Just as leaders mistakenly apply technical solutions to solve adaptive problems in their organizations[2], we make the same mistake when trying to achieve personal adaptive change. Simply resolving to follow a list of expected or ideal behaviors represents a technical solution that is unlikely to achieve our goal. There are underlying assumptions that motivate our secondary drivers that need to be addressed.

These unspoken assumptions are considered by us to be incontrovertible facts. We hold them as true, and we never challenge their validity. Each of us creates filters based on our underlying assumptions that allow us to process the world. And these filters protect us from challenges to our identity and to our

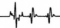

sense of personal well-being. They are the equivalent of the immune system for our ego. In many cases, this immune system becomes overactive and rejects new ideas and new ways of looking at the world[1]. Just as Mary's immune system became overactive and began attacking her blood vessels and nerves, the immune system of the mind can prevent us from growing and adapting to our increasingly complex world and can cause us harm.

To overcome our overactive mental immune system and bring about adaptive change, we have to stop looking through these filters and instead look at them. It is important to understand when and how these filters were derived and to carefully reexamine their viability under our current conditions. Nearly all of these unspoken assumptions originated at an earlier stage of our lives when they allowed us to adapt to our environment and helped us to succeed. Over time, if they are not reexamined and adjusted, these longstanding assumptions can impair our growth and interfere with our continued success. Therefore, when attempting to achieve personal adaptive change, we should add an additional column to our driver diagram, titled *underlying assumptions* (see **Figure 7.1**).

Returning to our hypothetical case, upon contemplating your underlying assumptions you realize that you are fearful of interacting with physicians because as a child you had a number of unpleasant experiences with a pediatrician, and you concluded that the best way to prevent being poked and prodded was to remain silent. This somewhat irrational assumption has never been directly confronted. Similarly, you now realize that your intrinsic shyness was an adaption to your childhood environment where your overbearing strict parents repeatedly warned that children should only speak when spoken to. And finally, you now realize that your eagerness to agree with others stemmed from an assumption that disagreement would result in a loss of popularity and friendship. Each of these assumptions needs to be challenged by actions and each action followed by self-reflection.

First you should attend the first meeting and plan to speak in response to the input of a physician on the committee. This action will create significant inward emotional stress, but it is unlikely to elicit a negative response on the part of any of the team members, including the physician. A self-reflective review of this data will allow you to question your underlying assumptions and encourage you to act again. By repeating the plan-do-study-act cycle several times, the emotional response to actions that contradicted your assumptions will gradually extinguish, and you will have corrected your overly active mental immune system and achieved a personal adaptive change.

Similar driver diagrams and plan-do-study-act cycles can be used to achieve other adaptive changes and allow all of us to continue to change and appropriately adjust to our environment. By undergoing personal adaptive change, we are better equipped to become adaptive leaders that can orchestrate transformational improvements in patient care.

Key Points about Immunity to Change
- Adults of all ages are capable of learning and increasing their mental complexity:
  - Neural plasticity persists for life; people can change!
  - New synapses and new neural connections can be constantly reconfigured.

- As we age, we create robust filters that block the input of discordant facts and ideas:
  - We need to look at rather than always look through these filters.
  - Our filters are analogous to an overly active immune system, and they prevent adaptation and can do us harm.

- We should use personal plan-do-study-cycles to breakdown our immunity to change:
  - We should examine the primary and secondary drivers that are interfering with our goals to make a behavioral or belief change.
  - Most importantly we need to
    - question the underlying assumptions that motivate our secondary drivers;
    - challenge these assumptions by action;
    - remember each challenge will cause emotional distress; and
    - know that with repeated challenge emotions dissipate and adaptive change is accomplished.

Action Plans for Nurses

Now that we understand that repetition is the key to learning, this section will summarize the key learning points of the five-point plan nurses can implement to bring about dramatic changes to how we deliver care in our hospitals and clinics. These are bold recommendations, and just as described in the example above, some nurses may be hesitant to act as a consequence of their immunity to change. When you hesitate, think of Mary's story and your own personal examples of patients who have been killed or injured unnecessarily. Each of us wants to think that the other guy will take care of these problems, but we all need to pitch in. This is every nurse's problem. Remember, many small steps add up to a very large step, but there can be no progress if we don't act.

Action Plans for Bedside and Clinic Nurses

What specific actions will be most strategic for nurses? Based on more than twenty years of analyzing and reanalyzing Mary's case and with the help of experts from many universities and many disciplines, as well as the assistance of Dina Treloar, ARNP, PhD—a close colleague who has worked with me for over fifteen years—I offer the following five point action plan for bedside and clinic nurses.

1. Understand and Apply Manufacturing and Athletic Principles in Your Day-to-Day Practice

Much of nursing requires physical motion, and motion studies have proved very helpful in reducing unnecessary walking and in searching for commonly used equipment. Industrial engineers can produce spaghetti diagrams that graphically depict wasted movement (see **Figure 2.5**), and these experts are being utilized in many medical centers. The ultimate goal of nursing systems improvements should be to maximize your presence at your patient's bedside. Geographically collocating your patients in adjacent rooms, placing commonly used reagents and equipment on small carts by the bedside, encouraging shift sign-outs at the bedside, and creating real time

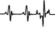

documentation systems that eliminate the requirement to take notes and batch reports at the end of each shift are some of the changes that can be instituted to allow you to devote the majority of your time to physically and emotionally caring for your patients.

When it comes to systems improvement, the nursing culture historically has encouraged workaround solutions to delivery system defects. Because many nurses lack psychological safety and are extremely busy, they have been hesitant to take their systems problems to the administrator that has the knowledge and authority to provide a permanent solution. When nurses continually utilize the same workaround solutions again and again to provide care for their patients, they eventually experience burnout[3].

For example, on an active medical floor in our hospital, nurses were responsible for monitoring the infection isolation carts to ensure they were stocked with isolation gowns. However, several times per day one or two of the carts ran out of gowns. Rather than notifying the supply manager, nurses chose to run down to the supply room and restock the carts, a job that was not assigned to them. By failing to create a permanent solution that ensured the supply administrator assigned an appropriate floor clerk to restock the gowns, each day the floor nurses were required to take time away from caring for their patients to work around this system defect and resupply the carts. To prevent these wasteful activities, all nurse supervisors need to monitor workaround solutions and assist floor nurses to create permanent systems solutions. They also should regard workaround solutions as a warning that nursing communication and job satisfaction require improvements.

Finally, all nurses should have a clear understanding of customer-supplier relationships. You are the hands-on caregiver for inpatient care, as well as for much of the routine follow-up care in the outpatient arena. You should realize that when it comes to physicians writing orders and providing instructions for care, they are your suppliers. You should expect clearly written, unambiguous orders and instructions that can be easily followed. If physicians are not fulfilling this role, they place both you and the patient in jeopardy. If orders or care instructions are not clear, it is critical that you ask specific questions to clarify your misunderstanding. Physicians should welcome these requests for clarification, and ideally they should apologize if their instructions were not sufficiently clear. Clear communication and coordination are critical conditions for any efficient, high-quality, and safe system.

> **Key Points about Using Manufacturing and Athletic Principles in Day-to-Day Practice**
> - Improve physical layouts to minimize motion and maximize time at the bedside.
>
> - Avoid workaround solutions, and be wary that they may lead to job dissatisfaction.
>
> - Understand customer-supplier relationships, and when it comes to orders and care instructions, physicians are the suppliers and you are the customer.

2. Actively Participate in Safety and Quality Initiatives

As a nurse you are truly on the front lines of care. Many of the defects in the systems of care directly impact you and your patients. A large percentage of preventable errors are associated with one of nursing's primary responsibilities: the administration of medications. As described in **Case 3.1**, when systems contain latent errors you are at risk of inadvertently hurting your patient. And depending on the safety culture of the institution, you are in danger of being blamed for an understandable and predictable human error[4]. Furthermore, you are at risk of becoming a second victim.

Because you know more about direct patient care than any other professional in the health care system, it is very important that you take an active role in quality and safety teams and become very familiar with PDSA cycles. You need to speak up and actively contribute to the planning cycle of all bedside care improvements, and you need to be involved in the piloting of these improvements before they are disseminated. In addition to being involved in improvements, you are in the ideal position to identify latent errors and to participate in failure mode and effects analysis (FMEA) to proactively prevent these potential errors from ever reaching your patients and your fellow nurses.

Because each FMEA requires the assembly of a team and is time consuming, Virginia Mason Medical Center has promoted another way of identifying errors and other system defects called patient safety alerts (PSAs)[5]. Too often when frontline health care providers detect problems, administrators ignore their complaints and may label the bearer of bad news as a troublemaker. This approach ensures that latent errors (the red beads) will never be removed, and the likelihood of patient injury will remain unchanged. At Virginia Mason, administrators are trained to immediately respond to all patient safety alerts. Each alert describes a medical systems defect, defined as any event that has the potential to jeopardize the safety or well-being of a patient. And each patient safety alert is graded[5]:

- Red events (1 percent of events)—these are life-threatening events, never-events, as well as any other conditions that have the potential to cause serious harm. Included in this category are actual or near misses, wrong-site surgery, accusations of sexual misconduct, disruptive behavior by staff or patients, and National Quality Forum reportable events including falls and grade 3–4 pressure ulcers.

- Orange events (8 percent of events)—these events are less severe, often involving interactions between different subspecialists or departments.

- Yellow events (91 percent of events)—these include any event felt to impede patient care or cause minor harm to patients, such as delays in patient transport, slow elevators, and stale food.

This program requires the full the support of administrators as well as physicians. However, when the safety climate is high and everyone is aligned in their desire to protect patients, you as the nurse can be invaluable in identifying and helping to eliminate errors and preventing patient injury. If your hospital system has a poor safety climate, with the help of fellow nurses, you can apply campaign techniques outlined in the previous chapter to improve your safety culture.

> **Key Points about Nursing Involvement in Safety and Quality Initiatives**
> - Nurses are directly impacted by systems that contain latent errors.
>
> - As frontline workers, nurses are in a position to identify errors and potential errors. They need to
>   - be active participants on all improvement teams and
>   - report all patient safety concerns, including
>   - high-risk events, and errors that cause serious injury;
>   - intermediate risk problems that interfere with coordination of care; and
>   - lower level events that interfere with the efficiency of care.

3. Actively Participate in Multidisciplinary Teams

Nurses are usually well trained in working within teams; however, during my observations of work rounds at five different medical centers, I discovered that most nurses are reticent to actively contribute data or opinions when physicians are present. Many admit to being intimidated. Too often physician-nurse interactions occur only when there is a problem or an error, and the negative feelings associated with these interactions often inhibit more routine interactions. Remember, you have a unique perspective and possess the greatest knowledge regarding your patient's recent complaints and emotional state. Your assessment of pain is particularly helpful, and when nurses and physicians share the same perspective regarding a patient's pain, there is less likely to be splitting on the part of the patient. Patients receiving narcotics for pain or simulating pain commonly set one caregiver off against another, claiming severe pain to one while demonstrating only modest pain to another. Because nurses observe patients over an extended period, they are able to accurately assess the true severity of a patient's pain, and they are the most capable of monitoring the benefits of pain medications.

By participating in work rounds, you will also be able to more accurately explain the medical team's management plans to your patients. You should also encourage your patients to actively participate in the medical team's deliberations. Active participation will increase your patients' understanding of their diseases and their motivation to adhere to treatments. Finally, because you will gain a better understanding of the team's management plans, you will no longer need to page team physicians to clarify their orders, providing you with additional time to interact and directly care for your patients.

Key Points about Nursing Participation of Multidisciplinary Rounds

- Actively participate on work rounds.

- Encourage patients to share their ideas and concerns on rounds.

- Have a full understanding of the management team's plans to reduce the need to page physicians for clarifications.

---

4. All Nurses Should Become Health Care Leaders

Nurses, unlike physicians, have no conflicts of interest when it comes to providing the most cost effective and safe care for their patients. As a nurse, you receive a fixed hourly salary for caring for your patients, not a fee for service. This makes you the ideal patient advocate, and because you spend the most hands-on time with patients, you have the best understanding of their needs and concerns. You are the ideal health care leader because your profession has never strayed from your primary mission to comfort and improve the health of your patients.

As health care undergoes profound system changes, your leadership will be very important. You must develop the courage to speak up on behalf of your patients. Safe medical cultures encourage a flattened hierarchy of power that provides the psychological safety that will allow you to contribute your unique perspective on each patient's medical and psychological needs. The development of checklists for intravascular device placement, as well as other procedures, are excellent tools for democratizing knowledge and allowing doctors, nurses, and patients to share the same information[6]. Checklists are very helpful tools not only for ensuring no step in an important procedure is overlooked but also for leveling the power gradient.

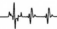

For example, in the comprehensive unit-based safety program (CUSP), nurses are required to "call out" when a physician breaks the sterile field or makes some other error while placing an intravascular device[7]. The physician is then obligated to correct his or her mistake. The important concept that both doctors and nurses need to embrace is that everyone makes errors. Both doctors and nurses must be willing and comfortable to second check each other's work. You should understand that the physician, just like every other human being, makes errors, and no single person will achieve perfection day in and day out. Only by utilizing systems with multiple second checks and other fail-safe designs can we hope to achieve perfection.

As a central member of the health care team, you should expect to be treated respectfully by those higher on the power chart, particularly physicians. Similarly, you should show mutual respect for those that assist you, including orderlies, transporters, janitors, and desk clerks. To establish a positive working environment that encourages joy at work, we all need to feel appreciated and respected.

Key Points about Nursing Leadership
- Nurses have no conflict of interest and are the ideal patient advocates.

- As leaders, you can protect the interests of our patients.

- You will benefit from a flattened power gradient:
    - Checklists allow nurses to second check physicians and vice versa.
    - You should expect and model mutual respect for all caregivers.

---

5. Campaign to Improve Your Hospital Systems' Culture of Safety

As nurses, you work throughout the hospital; nurses usually are not divided into separate departments like physicians. This condition happily eliminates problems with silos and distinct subgroups, making nurses the most united of all hospital system professionals. In my experience at multiple medical centers, I have repeatedly observed that nurses understand the hospital social environment far better than physicians and possess broader social networks. These conditions make you the ideal health system campaigner, and it is no coincidence that administrators often identify nurses as the lead professional group to initiate quality campaigns.

Lively twenty to thirty minute educational programs, role playing exercises, brochures, posters, and buttons can all supplement one-on-one interactions and other large group gatherings to improve adherence to safe practices and to improve morale. A number of successful campaigns led by nurses have been reported in medical journals, including dignity for all patients[8], hand washing[9], power for nursing[10], and health provider influenza vaccine campaigns[11]. The number of potential campaigns that nurses could initiate to improve defective processes and cultural deficits is infinite. The organizing techniques described in Chapter 6 have great potential to transform every medical center. And when it comes to encouraging passion and commitment to improve the care and safety of our patients, nurses can and should lead the way.

Key Points about Nursing Campaigns to Improve the Culture of Safety

- Nurses have a broad understanding of hospital system culture and have extensive social networks.

- They are ideal campaigners for cultural change.

Action Plans for Nurse Practitioners

Nurse practitioners as well as physician assistants play a unique and important role in modern health care. This section will focus on nurse practitioners; however, these suggestions also apply to physician assistants. These two classes of caregivers are often termed *physician extenders* because they allow the physician to appropriately utilize his or her higher-level training to manage the more complex iterative cases in which the diagnosis is uncertain or unexpected complications have arisen. As the industrial world's population ages, the burden of illness will increase, and there is projected to

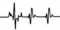

be a physician shortage. An effective way to compensate for this shortage will be to train more physician extenders.

1. Apply Key Manufacturing Principles to Your Practice

- *Customer-supplier relationships*—effective nurse practitioners have a clear understanding of their working relationships with their supervising physician or physicians. The nurse practitioner-physician customer-supplier relationship is one of the most complex in medicine because each party is both a customer and a supplier. In the case of the nurse practitioner, he or she is supplying assistance to the physician, and the physician as the customer should be happy with the care being provided and trust the expertise of the nurse practitioner. Similarly, the physician is supplying supervision and teaching to the nurse practitioner, and the nurse practitioner should be happy with the intellectual and emotional support of the physician. Together the nurse practitioner and the physician should decide which cases are most appropriately managed by the nurse practitioner and which cases are most appropriately managed by the physician. Over time and by trial and error, they can establish stable, effective triage and handoff protocols that will allow them together to provide the best possible care for their patients.

- *Understanding and improving value streams*—nurse practitioners are often called upon to manage patients requiring sequential care and therefore are in a unique position to improve patient care. Understanding and improving value streams has potential to reduce wasteful procedures and tests, and in the case of hospitalized patients, it could shorten hospital stays. You can incorporate the clinical guidelines from subspecialty and primary care societies into each patient value stream to ensure patients receive the most up-to-date and scientifically based care (see next page).

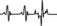

Case 7.1. Mrs. Smith is a seventy-year-old female, retired bank executive who was admitted to the hospital with complaints of intermittent fevers of 101°F for two months. Her fever was associated with mild muscle aches. However, her appetite was good, and she denied any weight loss. She also noted mild fatigue associated with her fevers. Other than a temperature of 101°F her physical exam was entirely normal. No lymph nodes were palpated, and her liver and spleen were of normal size on abdominal exam. She lives in New Haven, Connecticut, and had not traveled outside the Northeast in over fifteen years.

The admitting practitioner ordered a huge battery of blood tests, including a malaria smear, antibody titers for leptospirosis, brucella, Rocky Mountain spotted fever, Ehrlichia, Lyme disease, and dengue fever. He also ordered a large battery of expensive imaging studies, including head, chest, and abdominal CAT scans; a gallbladder ultrasound; and an indium-label white blood cell scan. The cost of her diagnostic workup was over $5,000.

All tests were negative. An infectious disease specialist was consulted to perform a complete history, including the past medical history. He learned that Mrs. Smith had suffered a seizure two and a half months earlier, which was thought to be secondary to a small stroke. She was started on Dilantin at that time, a medication that prevents seizures and induces fever as a common side effect. The consultant recommended discontinuing Dilantin and adding a different antiseizure medicine. Within seven days of discontinuing Dilantin, her fever resolved.

- *Reduce waste by effective decision making*—waste is a major problem when it comes to patient care, and experts estimate that 30 percent of our health care dollars are wasted[12]. Much of that waste is the consequence of poor decision making on the part caregivers. In many medical centers, those who manage patient care fail to make the hard

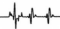

choices of picking the single most cost effective test or therapy. As described in **Case 7.1**, too often practitioners unthinkingly order a huge battery of tests on admission. They fail to recognize that illnesses like FUO are iterative in nature and cannot be managed using simple care protocols or algorithms. When in doubt they check off every possible test to explore the hundreds of causes for fever. A far wiser and cost-effective approach is to obtain a very complete history, perform a careful physical exam, and order a limited number of inexpensive tests to exclude dangerous diseases that would require immediate attention. For example, one the more dangerous causes of fever is sepsis or bacteria in the blood. Blood cultures should be drawn to quickly exclude this possibility, and blood cultures were negative in Mrs. Smith's case.

Once these basic screening procedures have been performed, the practitioner needs to apply Sutton's law. Willie Sutton was a famous bank robber who when captured was asked by reporters, "Willie, why do you rob banks?" Willie replied, "That's where the money is."[13] Clinicians should order tests and treatments that are likely to have a high yield. They need to go for "where the money is." In **Case 7.1**, based on Mrs. Smith's history, the admitting practitioner should have discontinued Dilantin before launching an expensive, low-yield diagnostic battery.

To achieve higher quality, safety, and efficiency, caregivers will be called upon to make the "right" diagnostic and therapeutic decisions for their patients. Unfortunately the majority of nurses, nurse practitioners, and physicians are never formally instructed in medical decision making, and a full discourse on this important skill is beyond the scope of this chapter. An excellent review of the subject is provided by the American College of Physicians' "Medical Decision Making."[14] Just as in **Case 7.1**, caregivers are frequently called upon to deal with uncertainty and are required to make an educated guess as to the true nature of a patient's illness.

When called upon to create a differential diagnosis as exemplified by **Case 7.1**, a complete history is of critical importance, and the practitioner who first managed Mrs. Smith failed to inquire about recent illnesses and medications. As the physician obtains the background data, he or she should be generating hypotheses, and then after the background data has been accumulated, he or she should generate additional questions, as well as choose laboratory and imaging studies that will confirm or refute the initial hypothesis. The usual steps recommended to systematically approach an unknown diagnosis are

1. generate alternative hypotheses;

2. gather data;

3. use the data to check the hypothesis; and

4. select a course of action:
    • order additional tests;
    • treat; or
    • wait for further manifestations.

Diagnostic tests most likely to identify "where the money is" need to be chosen carefully, taking into account pretest probability and post-test probability using Baye's theorem (see next page). If a disease is highly improbable before the test is ordered, a positive or negative test is unlikely to secure the diagnosis. This is the equivalent of Willie Sutton choosing to rob an orphanage! For example, in **Case 7.1**, ordering a malaria smear was a wasteful test because Mrs. Smith had no history of travel outside of Connecticut, and Connecticut has not had a case of endemic Malaria reported in more than one hundred years[15]. Given the exceedingly low prevalence of malaria in Connecticut (we will assume she had a remote possibility of contracting the disease from a mosquito that had bitten an infected traveler), the pretest probability for malaria was less than 0.01 percent.

A malaria smear has a true positive rate of approximately 90 percent and a false positive rate of 0.1 percent[16] (these values vary greatly depending on the expertise of the technician). Applying Baye's theorem, as shown below, the post-test probability after a negative malaria test is 0.1 percent, and after a positive smear only 8.2 percent. These probabilities would not alter the clinician's decision making.

Baye's Theorem

True Positive (TPR) = number of diseased patients with a positive test/ total diseased patients

False Positive (FPR) = number of undiseased patients with a positive test/total undiseased population (FPR)

Pretest probability (p[D])

Post-test probability (ptest [D])

Probability of disease when the test is positive

$$ptest\ [D] = \frac{p[D]\ x\ TPR}{p[D]\ x\ TPR + \{(1 - p[D])\ X\ FPR}$$

+ *Malaria smear calculation of post-test probability (**Case 7.1**)*

*.0001 x 0.9/0.001 x 0.9 + (1-0.0001) x 0.001 = **8.3%***

Probability of disease when the test is negative

$$ptest\ [D] = \frac{p[D]\ x\ (1 - TPR)}{p[D]\ x\ (1 - TPR) + \{(1 - p[D])\ X\ 1 - FPR}$$

Malaria smear calculation of post-test probability (Case 7.1)

*0.0001 x 1-0.9 = 0.00001/ 0.00001 + 0.9999 x 0.001 = **0.1%***

A key lesson can be derived from Baye's theorem: when disease prevalence is low, the probability of a false positive test is greater than the probability of a true positive test, and the test will not be of benefit. Similarly, if based on history, epidemiology and baseline laboratory testing, the probability is very high (85–95 percent range) then the addition of a confirmatory test will not result in a significant rise in the post-test probability of disease[14]. The practitioner should always ask, "How will a negative or a positive test result affect my decision making?" If the answer is not at all, as was true of the malaria smear, then the test should not be performed.

Based on our understanding of clinical problem solving, a practitioner requires 10,000 hours of experience in clinical care (forty hours a week clinical work would take four and a half years; twenty hours a week would take nine years) before he or she can achieve maximal expertise[17]. Clinicians need to be well schooled in the skills of differential diagnosis, hypothetical problem solving, Baye's theorem[14], and pattern recognition[18]. This last skill is most important for achieving a rapid diagnosis, and experts intuitively know "when everything adds up."[19] Intuitive pattern recognition is very helpful but should not be regarded as sufficient evidence to take action without additional objective evidence. Medical diagnosticians also need to be aware of many of the cognitive traps that can lead to misdiagnosis[14, 19], including the following elements:

- *Confirmation bias*—inappropriately assuming the patient has a common disease and ignoring the possibility of a less common disorder. This error can occur when the caregiver fails to ask open-ended questions and instead asks biased questions designed to confirm a specific predetermined diagnosis. Alternatively, inexperienced clinicians too often focus on a very rare disease when all the manifestations are also consistent with a common disease. In this circumstance probability would favor the common disease. "When you hear hoof beats, don't first think of zebras." Beware that

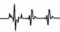

patients can distract you with diagnoses they read about or heard about from friends. It is important to take this information into consideration, but don't allow it to steer you in the wrong direction.

- *Commission bias*—taking action too quickly before the diagnosis has been clarified. Action-oriented caregivers need to be encouraged to use the tincture of time as a diagnostic tool in difficult cases. Often the illness takes time to declare itself through specific symptoms and signs. Action is only justified when one of the possibilities is a life-threatening disease.

- *Unwarranted certainty*—assuming that impeccable logic can create certainty. Practitioners need to express uncertainty to other team members and to their patients. Humility is an important characteristic that all caregivers need to embrace. Dogmatic certainty often leads to serious errors.

- *Culture of conformity*—nurses and physicians are susceptible to groupthink, and despite evidence in the literature and recommendations by professional subspecialty organizations to the contrary, they may continue local "traditional" approaches to specific diseases. Periodically it is critical to reexamine common practices. Also when cases are referred with a specific diagnosis from another hospital or care team, all clinical data should be viewed from fresh perspective, and the admitting diagnosis should be actively questioned.

- *Improperly weighting of data*—practitioners may overly focus on positive data and ignore important and relevant negative data. They can be overly influenced by single characteristic such as a past history of excellent health. Decisions can also be influenced by a negative attitude toward a patient. Patients who are not well spoken or who have poor hygiene or other less desirable attributes may receive poorer health care. I suspect this is often due to inadvertent stereotyping. We all must be careful to treat all of our patients equally, regardless of our own personal biases.

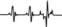

- *Satisfaction of search*—the act of discontinuing the search once a single disease is identified can lead to misdiagnosis. It is always important to create a broad differential and consider other possible etiologies before taking action.

- *Vertical line failure*—not being mindful of a less conventional possibility and not using lateral thinking. Practitioners should never accept the prevailing diagnosis, but rather they should attempt to reframe the problem whenever possible.

As discussed in Chapter 2, only 20 percent of medical cases are iterative in nature like **Case 7.1** and Mary's case. These cases represent diagnostic dilemmas that require differential diagnosis, hypothesis generation, and repeated cycles of testing to narrow uncertainty sufficiently to take action. Management of these patients is distinctly different from the 80 percent of patients that can be managed through sequential care that is guided by protocols or algorithms. To ensure efficiency and high quality, iterative-care patients should be managed by a separate team usually led by physician with a minimum of nine to ten years of experience in differential diagnosis, and the team should consist of highly experienced residents and nurses who are well schooled in medical decision making. This team can brainstorm regarding the possible underlying causes of each patient's symptoms and signs and design an efficient diagnostic strategy.

Once a diagnosis is confirmed, each patient should receive protocol-driven sequential care that is based on prior clinical studies, the guidelines of subspecialty national and international organizations, and Baye's theorem. A clearinghouse of diagnostic and therapeutic protocols is available through the Agency for Health Care Research and Quality (AHRQ, http://www.guideline. gov, accessed 1/3/11). Less experienced care teams can orchestrate these protocols, and the use of protocols can serve as an ideal mechanism for training new caregivers in the application high-quality, scientifically based approaches to known diseases. The use of protocols promises to improve the consistency of care, reduce the inappropriate use of unnecessary procedures, and reduce the expense of care. Furthermore, as team members gain greater familiarity with care protocols they will become capable of identifying patients who are not responding as expected. They can refer such nonresponders to an iterative management team to investigate other potential causes of their symptoms.

Key Points about How Nurse Practitioners Should Make Medical Decisions

- For diagnostic dilemmas, start with a complete history and physical exam and inexpensive screening laboratory tests and then
  - generate alternative hypotheses, gather data to check each hypothesis, and select a course of action;
  - use iterative testing to narrow uncertainty; and
  - apply Sutton's law (go for "where the money is").

- Use Baye's theorem to guide testing and to determine the pre-test and post-test probability.
  - If there is a low pretest probability or a high pretest probability of disease, don't order the test.

- Keep in mind, pattern recognition is used by experts, and maximal skill takes more than 10,000 hours of experience.

- Beware of cognitive traps: confirmatory bias, commission bias, unwarranted certainty, cultural conformity, improperly weighted data, satisfaction of search, and vertical line failure.

- Remember,
  - only twenty percent of cases are iterative and require experienced teams and
  - 80 percent of cases are sequential or algorithm driven and can be managed by novice teams.

---

2. Accept the Fact that We All Make Errors, and Embrace Safety and Quality Initiatives

Case 7.2. My wife Kathie was T-boned by a huge SUV in February of 2009. Fortunately, her side airbags deployed, and she survived the crash. She suffered five severely fractured ribs on her left side, as well as a ruptured spleen. Following surgery to remove her spleen, she was discharged on the fifth hospital day. Over the next two weeks, she continued to gain strength and began walking on her treadmill. However, she noticed she could only walk short distances before becoming short of breath. I noticed that she had to pause in midsentence to take a breath.

At our follow-up trauma clinic visit, Kathie described her shortness of breath, and I concurred. We wondered if she was excessively anemic or if there were any problems with her lungs. The physician assistant minimized her complaints and jokingly stated she seemed fine. I wasn't convinced by his reassurance. To appease my concerns, he listened to Kathie's lungs quickly and told us, "Her lungs sound fine. No need to see us again. She can go back to work when she feels up to it."

We were unhappy with his assessment and the next day Kathie saw her general internist, who upon her lung examination could hear no breath sounds in the area of the left lung. She ordered a chest X-ray and an hour later called us with the result: Kathie's entire left lung space was filled with fluid, and the lung had collapsed. No wonder Kathie was short of breath. She required hospital readmission and had more than three liters of bloody fluid drained from her left chest.

Case 7.2, like Mary's encounter with the neurologist, illustrates the consequences of distracted care. The physician assistant minimized Kathie's complaints of shortness of breath, performed a very cursory lung exam, and missed the finding of absent breath sounds throughout the left lung field (indicates fluid accumulation). Many of us hold the misconception that the majority of errors are the result of caregivers like the one described in this case. However, studies reveal that inattention and poor attitude explain only a small percentage of errors[20]. Certainly individuals who lack sufficient discipline and are lackadaisical in their approach to patients should be disciplined. However, as **Case 3.1** illustrates, more often well-meaning and conscientious caregivers are the victims of poor systems. As discussed earlier, errors are usually the consequence of bad systems and not bad people.

Nurse practitioners, nurses, and physicians all need to realize that humans make errors every day of their lives, and systems should be designed to compensate for this well-known trait. When in doubt, we should blame the system over the individual, and we should understand that if an error occurred once, it is highly likely to occur again and again unless the appropriate systems improvements are implemented. We need to understand that vigilance and trying harder will never allow us to reduce error rates below one out of one hundred. In order to achieve the levels of reliability required to prevent harm from reaching our patients, we will need to develop computer and automated machine forcing functions, checklists, and bundles. Once these are created, we should work to ensure that our colleagues adopt these critical tools for preventing human errors.

We should be ever mindful that variation is an intrinsic characteristic of everything we do in health care. Remember the red bead exercise, and utilize root cause analysis (RCA) and failure mode and effects analysis (FMEA) to remove latent errors whenever and wherever possible. Our efforts should be multidisciplinary and involve every level of the health care team. Most exciting, when we are continually looking for ways to improve quality and safety, our work becomes more challenging and more meaningful. Continual change is an underlying characteristic of evolution, and caregivers should assist our microsystems to evolve toward safer, higher quality, and more patient-centered processes. Remember patients see caregivers and the system of care as one. If our systems are defective, we are all in danger of being viewed as uncaring.

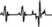

Key Points about How Nurse Practitioners Can Prevent Errors and Improve Quality

- Nurse practitioners should understand that everyone makes errors.
  - Errors can result from poor attitude; however, most errors are the consequence of bad systems.
  - Increased vigilance and trying harder are ineffective for preventing patient harm.
- Variability is a characteristic of all systems, and our job is to remove latent errors in order to improve reliability.
- Failure mode and effects analysis (FMEA) and root cause analysis (RCA) are effective methods to improve quality.
- Nurse practitioners should encourage and lead a multidisciplinary effort to improve our systems.

---

3. Teamwork Is a Necessity

The ability to work in teams is a necessity for nurse practitioners. Physician extenders by definition are always working in a team. Sometimes this will be a team of two, but more often you will be working in management teams consisting of more than one physician, several nurses, a pharmacist, and a case manager. As the nurse practitioner, you are in a unique position to encourage communication between nurses and physicians because you can understand both perspectives. You can encourage physicians to flatten the hierarchy of power to create a zone of emotional safety that will in turn encourage meaningful input by nurses. I have observed that when the treatment plans of nurses and doctors are aligned during work rounds, bedside nurses no longer feel the need to frantically page physicians or nurse practitioners to clarify their orders. My residents observed a greater than 50 percent reduction in pages[21].

Patients and patient families should be included as part of your team whenever possible. By truly partnering with them, you will improve commu-

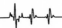

nication and increase trust. When patients are fully informed regarding the rationale behind each treatment plan, they are more likely to adhere to their treatments and more likely to express high satisfaction with your care.

By helping to nurture team identity, you can encourage team members to focus on their mutual goal—the best possible care for their patients—rather than focusing on their own individual needs and concerns. True team spirit has the potential to disseminate throughout the medical center, improving the culture of safety and enhancing the sense of community. By fostering true teamwork, you and your fellow caregivers can bring the joy back to health care.

> **Key Points about Nurse Practitioners and Teamwork**
> - Physician extenders are always part of a team.
> - Nurse practitioners can assist in integrating bedside and clinic nurses into the care team.
> - Nurse practitioners can help to lower the power gradient and thereby enhance the zone of safety.
> - Teams should include patients and patient families as part of the team.
> - Nurturing teamwork increases the focus on the patient and increases job satisfaction.
> - Teams have the potential to bring the joy back to health care.

4. Lead by Example

Although nurse practitioners serving as physician extenders will be under supervision, that does not mean they cannot be leaders. Nurse practitioners generally devote full time to the frontline management of patients and therefore are very familiar with the processes of care, as well as the impediments to care. Effective nurse practitioner leaders speak out about these impediments and can play a leading role in quality improvement teams. Secondly, nurse practitioners can lead by example because they are ever present on the wards and in the clinics and interact closely with every group of caregivers. By modeling respectful communication, friendliness, self-control, industriousness, enthusiasm, inquisitiveness, humility, honesty, and compassion, as a nurse practitioner, you can serve as an ideal role model for nursing and medical students as well as other caregivers.

Key Points about Nurse Practitioner Leadership
- Has a unique frontline perspective and should serve leadership roles on quality improvement teams

- Can lead by example by modeling ideal caregiver behavior

---

5. Serve a Unique Role in Campaigns to Change Health Care Culture

Just like bedside and clinic nurses, most of you have rich social networks, making you very effective campaigners. In addition you have close working relationships with physicians, and this will allow you to bring physicians into your campaigns. I have noticed in our hospital that physicians are reticent to join campaigns designed to bring about change, and they usually complain they are too busy. However, when approached by a close colleague with compelling personal narratives, physicians can be recruited into campaigns. If this constituency can be reached, the likelihood of true change throughout the health system is greater. So get out there and recruit your physician colleagues.

Key Points about Nurse Practitioners and Campaigning
- Nurse practitioners have broad social networks, which increases their effectiveness.

- Because of close working relationships, they have the potential to recruit physicians to a campaign.

Action Plans for Nursing Administrators

During Mary's illness, we never saw a single administrator. In fact, as a junior faculty member, I didn't know the name of single nursing administrator. Administration was invisible to the majority of physicians in our medical center, and I believe this condition in part explained the poor systems of care within the institution. I never blamed administrators because they were invisible. And I understand that many administrators see their roles as quietly supporting the mission of the medical center and "staying out of the way" of physicians. Based on my personal experience and my analysis of our problems, I recommend a new 5-point plan for nurse administrators that will increase their visibility to patients and greatly improve their effectiveness in bringing about true change on the front lines.

1. Manage from the Front Line, Not from the Office

Care of our patients takes place in the clinics and on the wards; it does not take place in the administrator's office. Therefore, shouldn't nurse, hospital, and clinic administrators spend significant time in the areas where the patients are being seen? Coaches of championship athletic teams remain on the sidelines of the field or floor where their athletes are playing.

Similarly, supervisors in successful manufacturing companies are situated close to their workers on the assembling line to allow them to come to the aid of their workers at a minute's notice.

For example, at Toyota manufacturing plants, whenever an assembly worker detects a defect in a car, he or she pulls a cord to notify their supervisor, and the supervisor arrives within thirty seconds to assist in the determining the cause and the best fix for the defect. If the supervisor and assembly worker together cannot solve the problem within a few minutes, the entire assembly line stops and other administrators quickly arrive on the scene to assist in problem solving[22]. The stopping of the assembly line prevents the production of additional defective cars. The error is contained, and the system is modified through rapid problem solving to ensure that the error never recurs.

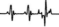

Shouldn't we in health care adopt this highly successful approach? Virginia Mason Medical Center has. When nurses, doctors, other caregivers, or clerks file a patient safety alert, an administrator takes responsibility to investigate immediately and creates a quick repair. For complex problems, the administrator is responsible for assembling an improvement team to create a more permanent solution[5].

Virginia Mason has also recently created job protocols for all administrators that designate specific times when each administrator will be physically present at a patient care delivery site. By being physically present, you as an administrator can speak directly to patients and assess their satisfaction, and you can also monitor the workflow of physicians and nurses. By gaining familiarity with the workforce and with each patient setting, you will be able to utilize your management skills to improve patient care far more effectively than sitting in a distant office simply managing by computer, performance bar graphs, and conference room conversations.

Another potential solution for establishing frontline management is the establishment of a unit-based leadership model consisting of a floor nurse leader, a physician leader, and an administrator (often a nurse) that together manage a discrete geographic location such as a floor, a clinic, or an intensive care unit[23]. Such frontline administrators can improve each unit's value streams by identifying roadblocks to care, problem solving, and working side by side with caregivers, clerks, and other support staff.

An excellent method for reconnecting you to your basic mission is to schedule a weekly breakfast meeting and invite any employee who has been hospitalized. During breakfast you should ask, "What rules did you need to break to make your care right?" These conversations quickly generate an improvement agenda and capture the true needs of our patients.

> **Key Points about Administrator Management on the Front Lines**
> - Administrators should be quickly available to manage safety alerts on the front lines.
>
> - A unit-based administrative structure keeps administrators physically present on the wards and in the clinics.
>
> - Breakfast meetings with employees who have been hospitalized will help identify operational barriers to care.

2. Focus on Improving Systems and Process Rather than Outcomes

Case 7.3. The clinicians throughout the system received the following email message:

> Good morning. Our hospital is at capacity, and we can no longer admit patients. Our emergency room is backed up with five patients requiring hospital admission, and there are nine patients in the holding unit. Please discharge your patients early today.

At the time of announcement, Mrs. M. was undergoing treatment for congestive heart failure. She was improving but continued to have some leg edema and required continued intravenous injections of a powerful diuretic (an agent that stimulates the kidneys to excrete water) to remove the residual body fluid.

After the email message, the senior physician caring for Mrs. M. decided that her diuretic treatment could be performed at home rather than in the hospital. He quickly discharged Mrs. M. to free up her hospital bed. He informed the case manager of his plan. As Mrs. M. was being taken by wheelchair to the hospital front entrance to be driven home, the case manager frantically called a home nursing company. The phone line was busy, requiring the case manager

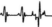

to quickly call a second visiting nurse service. Fortunately they answered, but they reported that a nurse would be unable to see the Mrs. M. for three days. Twenty-four hours later, Mrs. M. returned to the emergency room short of breath. Despite instructions given to her at the time of her discharge, she was unable to administer the intravenous diuretic, and her lungs had again filled up with fluid, causing her to become short of breath.

In his email, the administrator is understandably calling out for help. However, he was focusing on the outcome of systems and procedures that had failed to keep up with patient care demands. He was requesting another outcome: rapid discharge from the hospital. By focusing on this outcome, the administrator was encouraging workaround solutions that proved to be counterproductive. Although the desired outcome was temporarily achieved, the senior physician's quick fix proved harmful to Mrs. M.

Too often hospital administrators are primarily rewarded for monetary outcomes, overlooking the reality that profits are often driven by the quantity rather than the quality of care. Until more accurate performance measures for quality and safety are available, rewards should be provided for changes in processes and structures known to improve patient care, such as teamwork and cooperation, adaptive leadership, and evidence of patient-centeredness.

Of course money will always remain a critical concern, and all institutions must be fiscally responsible. However, improved processes and system structures promise to improve financial outcomes (see **Figure 7.2**). Athletic teams devote all their practice time to improving how they run each play, not on what the score will be. Similarly, manufacturing companies like Toyota focus on continually improving teamwork and technique on their assembly lines and on improving the systems that support the assembly line. They do this because they know that these improvements will yield a higher quality car built in a shorter period of time. And these outcomes in turn will yield higher profit margins.

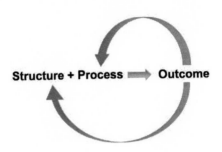

Figure 7.2. Relationships between structure, process, and outcome

Similarly, improved patient flow in hospitals and clinics will yield shorter waiting times and free inpatient beds for additional patient admissions. By focusing on the bottlenecks for patient flow, just as Southwest Airlines has been able to attain maximum value from their most expensive asset (their Boeing 737 planes), we can attain maximum value from our most expensive assets (our hospitals and outpatient clinics). We should avoid strictly focusing on outcomes, but rather we should utilize outcomes as feedback to determine if specific changes in process and structure are truly improvements.

Key Points about the Administrative Need to Focus on Process and Structure, Not Outcomes

- Focusing on outcomes can result in workaround solutions.

- Focus and reward process and structural improvements.

- Outcome should be used as the measurement to determine if changes in process and/or structure are true improvements.

---

3. Embrace and Reward Adaptive Leadership at All Levels

As discussed throughout this book, the prevention of cases like Mary's from ever occurring will require more than simple technical fixes. Profound changes in the way we do things will be necessary. We will need adaptive change, and adaptive change always generates anxiety. As previously discussed, whenever there is true adaptive change, there will be losers and there will be winners, and those who stand to lose are almost always those with the most power. Thus adaptive change is dangerous to those who are trying to lead.

If you as a nurse administrator wish to be an adaptive leader—a critical need in health care—it will be important for you to first obtain approval and understanding from those responsible for your supervision. They must understand your goals and strongly support them. You should warn them that your actions will create discord and that without emotional disequilibrium, you will be unable to achieve your agreed upon goals (see **Figure 5.3**).

If you are unable to garner strong support and a willingness to tolerate disequilibrium from those above you, then you should not undertake the proposed adaptive change (see **Figure 7.3**). Without administrative alignment, not only will you fail to make the changes you had planned, but you will also likely lose your job.

When adaptive change is initiated, those in favor of the status quo will attempt to reduce their discomfort by discrediting you as the instigator of the change. One of the best ways to counter this strategy is to assemble a leadership team to assist you in creating an effective strategy for enacting your changes. By diffusing the responsibility and continually sharing your ideas with like-minded supporters, you can maintain your perspective and avoid the traps of appearing self-righteous or overly zealous. Most importantly, you will no longer provide those in favor of the status quo with a single target for personal attack.

Alternatively, those who wish to preserve the status quo will delay the work required to bring about change, your goal will not be achieved, and those above you will perceive you as an ineffective leader. Some of the common idea killers you will hear include[24]: We tried that already; we've never done that before; we don't do it that way here; that never works; not in our budget; we don't have time; people won't like it; it's not part of your administrative responsibility. By creating a working team to assist you, you will be able design tactics to overcome these objections. There are a number of tools that can assist you in overcoming resistance to change. The tool kit designed by Rosabeth Moss Kanter of the Harvard Business School will be particularly effective, and applying the tool kit's ten practices will increase the likelihood of success (see **Figure 7.3**). The identification of champions, creating educational and training programs accompanied by action tools, as well as orchestrating quick-win pilot programs can all help to overcome resistance.

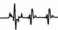

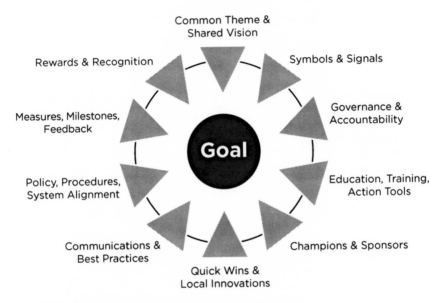

Figure 7.3. Rosabeth Moss Kanter toolkit for adaptive change
© Copyright 2011 by Rosabeth Moss Kanter, Harvard Business School. Used by permission. Excerpted from Kanter, "The Change Wheel: Elements of Systemic Change and How to Get Change Rolling," Harvard Business School Case 9-312-083, Harvard Business Publishing, Boston MA. An online version at www.reinventingeducation.org.

Administrators at the highest levels, including high-level nursing administrators, in our health care systems need to embrace adaptive leadership, and ideally they should become adaptive leaders. Alternatively it will be important that they understand adaptive leadership and help to manage the disequilibrium that naturally arises during true cultural change. Rather than relieving adaptive leaders of their duties because those below them are expressing unhappiness with change, they should understand that this is a manifestation of successful adaptive leadership.

A better course of action for high-level administrators is to advise the adaptive leaders and assist them in creating strategies to minimize personal attacks and work avoidance. In many cases, higher-level administrators can run interference by establishing milestones for changes that are accompanied by awards, reiterating the goals of change, and governing by accountability. Every leader should expect loyalty to the institution and acceptance of its common goals. And everyone should understand that those who continually obstruct meaningful change are by their actions disloyal to the institution and its mission. If we hope to achieve a culture of safety and quality and create the systems of patient care we aspire to, administrators will need to acknowledge that it is the obstructionist and not the adaptive leader who is the problem. We should be rewarding those who are leading change rather than rewarding the defenders of the status quo by dismissing those who favor change.

Key Points about Administrators Who Lead Adaptive Change

- It is important to first secure alignment of higher-level administrators.

- You should create a leadership team to assist with strategy and diffuse resistance.

- You should utilize champions, educational, and training programs combined with action tools and quick win pilot programs to overcome resistance to change.

- Higher-level administrators should support adaptive leaders by creating milestones and rewards, reiterating the goals of change, and governing by accountability.

---

5. Encourage and Practice Transparency

Transparency on the part of both caregivers and administrators is a critical component of a culture of safety, and we should all embrace the right of our patients to be fully informed about their care and any errors in delivery. Without transparency, trust quickly dissipates. When patients no longer trust their physicians, nurses, and administrators, they are far more likely to seek outside legal intervention. Patients are our stakeholders, and they are investing in our care system. As stakeholders they deserve full disclosure regarding both our successes and our failures.

What do we mean by transparency, and how do we achieve it? As Midwesterners, my parents encouraged us to always tell the truth. They repeatedly said, "Truth is always the best policy." As a naïve adolescent, I was saddened by the realization that many of my classmates, and even some of those in charge, did not subscribe to this policy. As a medical student and resident, I assumed that physicians and administrators would always search for the truth and that we should "tell it like it is and not how we wanted it to be." Again I was disappointed.

With advent of the Internet, Twitter, YouTube, texting, and multicopy email, we are approaching an era of true transparency; as never before, the truth promises to prevail. Given this reality, many hospital administrators are beginning to open their books and truly share their performance with the public. Hospital-hospital comparisons of patient satisfaction, appropriate use of antibiotic prophylaxis for surgery, readmission rates for congestive heart failure, and percentage of patients receiving effective treatment for pneumonia can be acquired with the click of a computer mouse (http://www.hospitalcompare.hhs.gov/ , accessed 1/7/11). It is only a matter of time before all hospital-associated complications and errors are publically reported.

We need to understand that our patients as stakeholders are unlikely to abandon us if we share our failures in addition to our successes. Patients and patient families can and should be our allies in our quest to improve quality, and they should be included on hospital boards, on quality improvement teams, and in root cause analysis determinations.

Many fear that the full disclosure of errors will increase the risk of litigation. However, Virginia Mason's experience proves otherwise. They have found that one out of eight patients suffering a fully disclosed error sues[5]. When patients are provided with a full explanation, receive a heartfelt apology from the physician as well as a high-ranking administrator, and are provided with the hospital's plan for preventing a recurrence of the error, patients are far less likely to sue.

When something goes wrong, the administration needs to declare that it happened; it shouldn't have happened; and it won't happen again[24]. The institution of an openness policy resulted in a 26 percent reduction in Virginia Mason's malpractice liability insurance expenses from 2007–2008, and these expenses continue to decline while the cost of malpractice premiums for other nearby institutions that continue their policy of secrecy continue to climb[5].

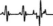

All nurses should also be encouraged to openly communicate. By creating a culture that blames the systems of care rather than the individual, nurses will feel safe reporting their errors, and rapid reporting will allow you as an administrator to rapidly contain the error. By instituting a quick fix, you can prevent a similar error for the immediate future and provide time for a multidisciplinary team to design a permanent correction. We will need to accept the reality that until our systems of care have been markedly improved, human errors will result in patient injury, and pushing these errors under the rug fails to mitigate and instead amplifies their harm.

Many of the strategies and tactics described in Chapter 6 for organizing people to bring about cultural change can be utilized to encourage transparency. During the coming decade, this issue promises to come to the forefront as patients become less complacent and more active, knowledgeable consumers.

Key Points about Administrative Transparency

- Patients are the hospital systems stakeholders, and they deserve full disclosure regarding their treatment and errors in care.

- Open disclosure, a heartfelt apology, and proof of a plan to prevent the reoccurrence of errors reduce the likelihood of a malpractice suit.

- Disclosure has reduced malpractice premiums at Virginia Mason Health Center.

- Nurses should be encouraged to disclose all errors so they can be contained.

- Hospitals should encourage a culture of openness, not blame.

Action Plans for Nursing Students

Our nursing schools and other health professional schools are now populated with a predominance of students from the millennium generation (born between 1982–2000). Many demographers now claim that this generation most resembles the last great generation who fought in World

War II[25]. Unlike the baby boomers or generation X who rebelled against their parents, the millennium generation identifies with and often follows the advice of their parents. As opposed to the baby boomers who demanded unconditional amnesty and were afforded excessive freedom to rebel, the millennials have grown up in a far stricter "zero tolerance" environment. They understand and embrace the rules of society.

They are not the typical self-absorbed youth of which most of us think, but rather they are usually cooperative team players who have worn school uniforms; played on youth soccer, volleyball, and basketball teams; and participated in community service. They were doted on by their parents and often received trophies for simply participating. As a group they are optimistic, idealistic, tolerant, and multicultural. Accompanying their idealism is a desire to have a meaningful job and to understand the rationale behind every action. They have high expectations of their leaders and see many of their parents' generation as hypocritical.

As a parent of two millennium generation children and having always lived by and espousing these same values, I am optimistic for the future of health care. My hope is that many of the barriers to improving patient care will be overcome by this remarkable generation, and it is the duty of those who are training this next generation of health care providers to build on their many strengths. Today's health professional students have the potential to greatly improve our systems of care, and by following the five recommendations listed below, they will be able to accelerate change.

Key Points about the Millennium Generation
- Predicted to be our next great generation
- Comfortable with authority and accepting of society's rule
- Cooperative and team oriented
- Desire meaningful jobs and want to make a difference in the world
- Optimistic, tolerant, and multicultural

---

1. Understand and Apply the Principles of Manufacturing and Athletics

Most nursing students choose their profession because of a desire to help people, a wish to give something to mankind, and a desire to save lives[26]. Many also naturally have a desire to be gainfully employed, but in general they are not oriented toward business or manufacturing. As a student, you may feel these disciplines have no relation to nursing; however, as discussed in Chapter 2, many of the best practices of companies like Toyota, Southwest Airlines, and Publix Supermarkets can and should be applied to health care. Therefore either during your undergraduate or postgraduate course work, you should attain a fundamental understanding of process protocols and system design, as well as customer-supplier relationships, the importance of continual feedback, and the generation of hypothesis-driven improvement.

As part of the millennium generation you are comfortable with change and with technology. Electronic records, electronic ordering, and electronically managed medication delivery and resupply are all quickly becoming standard operating systems within our health care systems. These electronic systems have the potential to improve care, but they will never take the place of face-to-face interactions, as so clearly exemplified by the ground crew coordinators of Southwest Airlines. As you become familiar with systems, you may be able to help design improvements that will ensure that caregivers never lose sight of their primary purpose comforting our patients and bringing them back to health. This cannot and should not be accomplished simply by sitting at a computer screen.

As electronic tools become more portable, the ability of carrying these tools to the bedside will allow more efficient documentation and sharing of information with your patients. Our goal should be to design computerized tools that increase the time caregivers are able to spend at the bedside and in the clinics, interacting face-to-face with patients.

> **Key Points about Student Learning about Industry and Athletic Principles**
> - Understanding and applying the best practices of Toyota, Southwest, Publix, and other companies can guide medical systems improvements.
>
> - Electronic tools may be helpful, but beware of reducing patient face-to-face time.

2. Become an Expert in Medical Decision Making

In nearly all health professions schools, including nursing schools, the acquisition of biomedical facts is emphasized. This approach ignores the fact that medical knowledge is continually changing, and many of the facts memorized today will be obsolete within five to ten years. A far more effective approach would be to emphasize understanding, encourage the thoughtful collection and analysis of data, and teach students how to effectively deliver care. Sadly in the United States only 55 percent of adult patients are receiving the recommended care that they deserve based on objective biomedical science[27]. What this finding tells us is that simply learning the facts does not translate into action. Not only do caregivers neglect to do the right thing, they often chose instead to order unnecessary tests and overtreat their patients.

Much of the undertreatment and overtreatment are the consequence of poor medical decision making, and nursing students—particularly those who aspire to be nurse practitioners—need to be schooled in the logical approach to making medical decisions based on probability and the generation of testable hypotheses. Nurses and nurse practitioners will benefit from training in differential diagnosis and applying probability to testing and decision making, because as patient management becomes more team oriented, nurses will be encouraged and expected to suggest possible diagnoses.

A summary of the basic approach to medical decision making is included in the action plans for nurse practitioners. Several important points should be emphasized for students. Effective differential diagnosis requires pattern recognition, and to achieve maximum pattern recognition skills requires 10,000 hours of experience[17]. Too often nursing students spend excessive time during their ward rotations listening to didactic lectures or reading. To become an expert, you will need to be actively involved in the diagnostic and treatment decisions for all the patients on your team. By suggesting possible diagnoses and putting your reputation on the line, you will learn from your mistakes far more than from your successes. Whatever the outcome of your suggestions, if you faithfully produce a differential diagnosis for every patient you encounter, you will progressively improve your diagnostic skills. Just as in mathematics, differential diagnosis is learned by practice, practice, and more practice.

In addition to learning how to create and test differential diagnostic lists, students need to understand and apply Baye's theorem to achieve cost-effective diagnostic testing, and this approach is also covered in the action plan for nurse practitioners. Several very simple rules should be kept in mind. If prior to ordering a test, everyone on your team feels the probability of the disease being tested for is extremely low, a positive test will not be helpful in significantly increasing the post-test probability, and the test should not be ordered. If the pretest probability of a specific disorder is extremely high, then ordering a confirmatory test is of no benefit because if the test is positive, it will not significantly improve the post-test probability of disease. Whenever the team is ordering a test, remember to ask, "How will a positive or a negative result affect how Ms. Jones is managed?" If the answer is that it won't, then you should encourage the team to refrain from ordering the test.

Key Points about Students and Medical Decision Making
- In addition to memorizing biomedical facts, students need to learn differential diagnosis including hypothesis generation and testing.

- Expertise in pattern recognition requires continual patient exposure and active problem solving.

- Cost-effective diagnostic testing requires an understanding of Baye's theorem.

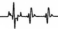
3. Learn and Understand the Principles of Reliability and Patient Safety

The majority of students only receive training in conventional statistics that encourage the grouping of data rather than following data over time. In the view of many safety experts, Deming's red bead experiment, run charts, and control charts should be required curriculum for all health professions students because you will all encounter the effects of excessive variability (too many red beads). And the lack of reliability in our care systems endangers our patients and increases the risk of you becoming a second victim. By understanding variability as well as the natural tendency for the human brain to make errors, you will realize that simply trying harder and increasing your vigilance will not prevent patient harm. You should be familiar with and utilize the tools that can reduce errors, including plan-do-study-act (PDSA) cycles, root cause analysis (RCA), failure mode and effects analysis (FMEA), checklists and bundles, computer order sets, and forcing functions. Many additional tools and educational programs are available through IHI Open School (http://www.ihi.org/IHI/Programs/IHIOpenSchool/, accessed 1/10/11), and every health professions school should create an IHI Open School chapter.

Key Points about Student Education in Quality and Safety

- The red bead experiment, run charts, and control charts should be required lessons for health profession schools.

- Students should understand random variation, reliability, and human error.

- Students should be able to apply the tools of safety PDSA cycles, RAC, and FMEA.

- Students should be encouraged to join IHI Open School.

---

4. Learn How to Effectively Work in Teams

Fortunately, team learning and team sports have played major roles in the upbringing of the millennium generation. However, teamwork in medicine promises to be more demanding, require a more complicated playbook, and require a sophisticated understanding of group dynamics. Because your generation truly wants to make a difference, it will be important that you agree as a group upon compelling goals for your team and keep them in the forefront even when you are exhausted and anxious during your training. Regard the principles of patient care as the Olympic Flame, representing the ideals of earlier nurses like Florence Nightingale (helped to reform the British Health System), Clara Barton (founder of the Red Cross), and Mary Eliza Mahoney (the first African American Registered Nurse and the cofounder of the American Nursing Association). You have chosen a wonderful profession, and you should continually remind yourself that your primary role is to learn how to comfort and heal the sick.

Your ability to level hierarchical power gradients and to communicate and work with authority figures will serve you well in modern nursing. Your willingness to collaborate is a great strength. However, beware of groupthink. Disagreeing with a management decision does not reflect poor teamwork. Without disagreements and a certain degree of creative abrasion, the true power of the team to generate new and more effective solutions will not be realized. Your willingness to be inclusive and to be open to others ideas also will prove of great benefit when working in teams. However, keep in mind that including too many members on your team will lead to process loss and decreased effectiveness. Recognize that all effective teams must have boundaries regarding who is on the team.

Your acceptance of rules and structure will also be of benefit when working on teams, and it will be important for you to learn how to establish sufficient structure to allow each team to accomplish their work but to avoid creating excessive structure that can stifle creativity and the joy of working on a team. And just as on your sports teams, you should expect your team

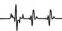

to be periodically coached. Self-coaching by periodically asking, "What went well, and what could be improved?" will also help you be part of ever improving teams.

Recognizing the importance of teamwork with physicians and pharmacists as well as other health professions, you should insist that your nursing school provide interdisciplinary team training. Simulation exercises with students from these other professions are one effective approach. The institution of a pass-fail grading system serves to reduce individual competition and encourages the formation of learning teams. In some professional schools, students are being formally assigned to learning teams for a semester, a year, or even the duration of their schooling. An increasingly popular system for learning called Team-Based Learning (TBL) has proven not only to be an effective format to learn specific facts and understand important concepts but also to teach teamwork. TBL requires a team launch, creates an ideal team structure, establishes norms for team behavior, encourages team spirit, and allows students to learn by teaching their fellow team members—all under the supervision of an expert facilitator[28].

Upon arriving on the clinical wards, your ability to work interdependently with others on your team will allow you to significantly contribute to the care of your patients because in the ideal team, all members will be expected to participate in management discussions. Armed with a rich understanding of team dynamics, you can assist other team members in assessing the effectiveness of your team and make suggestions on how your team can improve. And as your team becomes more and more effective, the care provided to your patients will become more efficient, safer, and higher quality. By your actions, you will be contributing to the improvement of your medical center's culture of safety and quality.

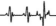

> **Key Points about Student Participation on Teams**
>
> - Keep your primary goal as a team member in mind: learning to comfort and heal the sick.
>
> - Beware of groupthink; creative abrasion makes for a productive team.
>
> - Keep your teams bounded because too many members reduce effectiveness.
>
> - Create enabling structure, and expect coaching.
>
> - Insist on the addition of teamwork training as part of your school curriculum.
>
> - Pass-fail encourages the formation of learning teams.
>
> - Team-base learning (TBL) can effectively teach teamwork as well as enhance learning.

5. Understand and Embrace Adaptive Leadership and Campaign for Change

As the newest members of the health care system, you should embrace your role as agents of change. You have no stake in the status quo, and after reading this book, you now realize that the status quo is harming our patients and is extremely inefficient. You will need to help eliminate the waste that clearly exists in our systems of care in order to prevent health care costs from progressively consuming our gross domestic product. To bring about change, you too will need to become adaptive leaders. Adaptive change could be dangerous as well as difficult for you as an individual student, because you are lowest on the totem pole of authority. But unlike older caregivers, you have a very large network of fellow students through classes, social activities, Facebook, Twitter, text messaging, and email. Your many contacts will prove very helpful in organizing campaigns for change. By creating leadership teams, you will be able practice your leadership and teamwork skills, and these skills will be benefit you not only during your campaigns but also during your

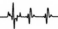

clinical training and in practice as a licensed caregiver.

Many social movements have been driven primarily by the youngest generation, and based on the assessment of demographers, you have the ideal traits required to improve our systems of care. You need to continually ask why, and when you don't like the answer, you should create a compelling campaign to bring about a change. Each campaign must be carefully designed to be modest in scope and to have a measurable and readily achievable goal. Campaigns are fun, and campaigns can truly improve our health care culture and change the way we do things. So get out there and change the world. I will be cheering you on.

Key Points about Student Adaptive Leadership and Campaigning
- Student adaptive leaders should ally with fellow students.

- Students have large social networks ideal for organizing campaigns to improve quality and safety.

- Campaigns with leadership teams provide excellent leadership and teamwork training .

- Students should ask why. And if they don't like the answer, they should consider organizing a campaign to bring about change.

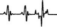
References

1. R. Kegan, and L.L. Lahey. 2009. *Immunity to Change: How to overcome it and unlock the potential in yourself and your organization.* Boston, MA: Harvard Business Press.

2. Ronald A. Heifetz, Alexander Grashow, and Martin Linsky. 2009. *The practice of adaptive leadership : tools and tactics for changing your organization and the world.* Boston, Mass.: Harvard Business Press.

3. A. Tucker, and A. Edmondson. 2003. Why Hospitals Don't Learn from Failures: Organizational and Psychological Dynamics That Inhibit System Change. *California Management Review* 45:55-72.

4. M. Green. 2004. Nursing Error and Human Nature. *Journal of Nursing Law* 9:37-44.

5. C. Kenney. 2010. *Transforming Health Care: Virginia Mason Medivcal Center's Pursuit of the Perfect Patient Experience.* New York, NY: CRC Press.

6. B. D. Winters, A. P. Gurses, H. Lehmann, J. B. Sexton, C. J. Rampersad, and P. J. Pronovost. 2009. Clinical review: checklists—translating evidence into practice. *Crit Care* 13 (6):210.

7. P. J. Pronovost. 2010. We need leaders: The 48th Annual Rovenstine Lecture. *Anesthesiology* 112 (4):779-785.

8. J. Clark. 2010. Defining the concept of dignity and developing a model to promote its use in practice. *Nurs Times* 106 (20):16-19.

9. E. E. Gillespie, F. J. Ten Berk De Boer, R. L. Stuart, M. D. Buist, and J. M. Wilson. 2007. A sustained reduction in the transmission of methicillin resistant Staphylococcus aureus in an intensive care unit. *Crit Care Resusc* 9 (2):161-165.

10. J. Sprinks. 2010. Developing nurses' power to care. *Emerg Nurse* 18 (1):12-15.

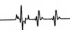

11. T. Ballestas, S. P. Mcevoy, and J. Doyle. 2009. Co-ordinated approach to healthcare worker influenza vaccination in an area health service. *J Hosp Infect* 73 (3):203-209.

12. D. Cutler. 2010. Analysis & commentary. How health care reform must bend the cost curve. *Health Aff (Millwood)* 29 (6):1131-1135.

13. R. G. Petersdorf, and P. B. Beeson. 1961. Fever of unexplained origin: report on 100 cases. *Medicine (Baltimore)* 40:1-30.

14. H. C. Sox, M.A. Blatt, M.C. Higgins, and K.I. Marton. 2007. *Medical decision making*. Philadelphia, PA: American College of Physicians.

15. C. W. Chamberlain. 1881. Malaria in Connecticut. *Public Health Pap Rep* 7:174-185.

16. C. Ohrt, W. P. O'meara, S. Remich, P. Mcevoy, B. Ogutu, R. Mtalib, and J. S. Odera. 2008. Pilot assessment of the sensitivity of the malaria thin film. *Malar J* 7:22.

17. Malcolm Gladwell. 2008. *Outliers : the story of success*. 1st ed. New York: Little, Brown and Co.

18. ———. 2005. *Blink : the power of thinking without thinking*. 1st ed. New York: Little, Brown and Co.

19. Jerome E. Groopman. 2007. *How doctors think*. Boston: Houghton Mifflin Co.

20. E. S. Fisher, J. P. Bynum, and J. S. Skinner. 2009. Slowing the growth of health care costs--lessons from regional variation. *N Engl J Med* 360 (9):849-852.

21. F. S. Southwick. 2010. Unpublished observations. Gainesville, FL.

22. J.K. Liker, and D. Meier. 2006. *The Toyota Way Field Manual*. New York, NY: McGraw-Hill.

23. V. Rich, P.J. Brenan, K. Williams, E. Riley-Wasserman, and L. May. 2008. Clinical leadership on the unit and at the top— a "Swiss Army knife" for sustained performance. Paper read at University of Pennsylvania Health System Consortium, Qualtiy and Safety Fall Forum, at Philadelphia, PA.

24. F. D. Loop. 2009. *Leadership and Medicine.* Gulf Breeze, FL: Fire Starter Publishing.

25. N. Howe, and W. Strauss. 2009. *Millennials Rising: The next great generation.* New York, N.Y.: Vintage eBooks.

26. J. Mcharg, K. Mattick, and L. V. Knight. 2007. Why people apply to medical school: implications for widening participation activities. *Med Educ* 41 (8):815-821.

27. E. A. Mcglynn, S. M. Asch, J. Adams, J. Keesey, J. Hicks, A. Decristofaro, and E. A. Kerr. 2003. The quality of health care delivered to adults in the United States. *N Engl J Med* 348 (26):2635-2645.

28. L. K. Michaelson, M. Sweet, and D.X. Parmelee. 2008. *Team-based Learning: Small Group Learning's Next Big Step.* Edited by M.D. Svinicki. Vol. 116, New Directions for Teaching and Learning. San Francisco, CA: Jossey-Bass.

—8—

FINAL THOUGHTS

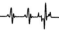
I hope this book has given you a great deal to think about. Is your head spinning? Do you feel overwhelmed by the challenges and new skills all health care providers need to acquire? If the problems were simple and represented technical fixes, they would have been solved by now. Caregivers would be working harmoniously together, all latent errors would have been eliminated from our care systems, carefully designed protocols based on established clinical scientific studies would be universally embraced, our leaders would be constantly exploring new ways to improve how we do things, and we would all be part of a culture that values our patient's interests above all else. Wouldn't it be exciting to know that when a patient walks into our clinic or hospital, they could enter our halls ensured that they would receive reliable, consistently safe, high-quality, cost-effective care that truly focuses on their health needs?

Our problems and our health care delivery systems are extremely complex. Just like Mary was, these systems are presently critically ill. However, just as in Mary's case, these systems can be cured. There will be no quick fix, and no one single leader can hope to solve the myriad of challenges we caregivers now face. As is true of all complex systems, improvements will need to occur simultaneously on multiple fronts. Understanding manufacturing and athletic principles will help, and understanding the nature of human error and the principles of quality and safety will also be of benefit. However, if I had to pick one area that I believe is most integral to improving how we care for patients, I would choose teamwork. If nurses, physicians, administrators, case managers, pharmacists, and other support personnel could work together and create an interdependent synergy, we could overcome many of our systems challenges. By checking our egos at the door and truly communicating seamlessly at all levels, the potential for improvement and change would be limitless.

If nurses can apply the tools described in this book to create new ways of doing things, the future for health care can once again become bright. We will be able to effectively implement the miraculous and innovative treatments brought to us by modern biomedical science. Imagine having a perfect day in the clinic or on the wards. All your patients are smiling and profusely thanking

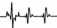

you for your effective and heartfelt care. No patient is required to sit in the waiting room or left on a stretcher waiting to be seen. Every medicine is given at the right dose and at the right time. Every patient receives only the tests and therapies they require to get well. All diseases are managed quickly and effectively, reducing human suffering and enhancing quality of life. Some say these goals are impossible and would represent true miracles.

But I believe these goals are achievable. They will not come as a single dramatic step but rather as many small seemingly trivial steps made by every caregiver. If we can consistently apply each tool to gradually but steadily improve our systems of care, one day we will achieve our goals. But we will never be able to rest on our laurels; that is the nature of quality improvement. Systems can always be improved, always be made more reliable and safer. I hope that after reading this book you will join me on the journey of continual improvement. My journey, like yours, is just beginning, and this book serves as the formal kickoff of my personal campaign to prevent other patients from experiencing the needless errors and poorly coordinated systems of care that nearly killed Mary.

INDEX

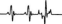

CPSIA information can be obtained at www.ICGtesting.com
Printed in the USA
BVOW020841250412

288623BV00001B/1/P